TAROT-CHI™

An Exercise System in 22 Forms

By

Shanna Warner

Tarot-Chi: An Exercise System in 22 Forms

Cover design, poses and artwork
By Mark Warner

Shanna Warner developed this exercise system.
No single Tarot deck inspired this system or book.
You do not need to have or own a Tarot deck to learn this exercise system.
Please consult with your physician before beginning.

For more about this book, visit: www.tarot-chi.com
Or my website: www.shannawarner.com

Published in 2021 by: Manna Services Group, LLC
Tulsa, Oklahoma

Print ISBN- 978-1-953098-07-8
E-book ISBN - 978-1-953098-08-5

This book is lovingly dedicated to my husband, Mark.
Thank you for believing in me and in this project.
And thanks for doing the exercise with me. It is more fun together.

CONTENTS

INTRODUCTION

How I came to be a fan of the Tarot.

"There are more things in heaven and earth, Horatio, than are dreamt of in your philosophy." - Shakespeare's Hamlet

WHEN I FIRST came across a deck of Tarot cards, I was a young woman in my 20s. I was out of college and graduate school, newly married and living in the big city. I was also a trauma survivor. So, I was open to anything positive that could help me reduce stress and feel better.

I was in a dusty, used bookstore. You know the kind - one where you are as likely to find a tattered copy of *The Anarchist's Cookbook* hidden on some shelf in a back room, as you are to find a Danielle Steele or Steven King paperback. There was a little bit of everything in that store, including several books about Tarot in the "Self-Help" section. One of the books had an unopened deck included. Hmmm? The package featured some lovely Art Nouveau designs, so I bought it.

The cards made an immediate impression on me. The artwork was beautiful! That is one of the things I love about Tarot decks - the visual impact and artistic beauty is enough to collect many decks. You can find decks dedicated to animals, real and imagined. You can find decks dedicated to art, modern and ancient. You can find decks dedicated to earth-based religions or even to Tolkien's *The Lord of the Rings*. But there is far more to Tarot than just fantastic art.

Most Tarot users believe the cards are linked to astrological, Egyptian, and Kabbalistic esoteric knowledge. (This book is not about that.) Some Tarot users believe the hidden knowledge should only be available to secret societies, with acolytes being taught in hushed ceremonies. (This book is not about that, either.)

We will not be delving into all the traditions of Tarot or discussing when and how it was created. We will not be talking about who has the better interpretation or the many levels of symbolism in any given deck. Those subjects have already been written about by scholars and mystics who are absolutely brilliant. I am not that scholar.

Instead, in *this* book, we will be using the Tarot as our inspiration to get moving physically! I will teach you my easy and effective exercise system based on the energy (chi) and images (archetypes) of the Tarot.

Energy. It is around us and inside us. Our body runs on electrical energy impulses, from the synapses in your brain to the beating of your heart. And our Earth itself is full of energy.

The metal core of our planet rotates and creates electrical currents of energy which create our magnetic poles. And all this energy is invisible! (Except when you see lightning or the aurora borealis.) An infinitesimal number of electrons, protons, neutrons and all manner of charged particles are inside and outside of you, they make the building blocks of YOU.

You are a creature of energy! Even ancient man knew this in a primitive way. Early human societies created stories to explain our energetic connections with the heavens and the Earth. These are the mystical stories of early man. The energy is invisible and the stories and ideas are ancient, but still real.

Since we are creatures of energy, we are going to use the energy of the archetypal images of the Tarot to balance and exercise our body! This exercise system is not physically difficult, but it is possible to get your heart rate up and break a sweat. If you need the support, you can stand and use a chair to hold onto for balance. You can also do the exercises while seated, making this a great system for older adults.

The Eastern world has long had traditions of physical exercise using the mental and psychological imagery of their world. Think of the various forms and poses taught in Yoga, Kung Fu, Tai Chi, or any of the martial arts. All are based in the mysticism of the Eastern world. All teach about the hidden energy fields (chi) in our bodies and our environment.

While I was taking martial arts classes, my thoughts always kept coming back to the imagery of the Tarot. My son learned Taekwondo and my late husband was a Wushu Master. They convinced me to take some classes. I loved it. But as my instructors were telling me to think of Yin and Yang, I kept thinking of Emperor/Empress, Fool/Universe, or other dualities and symbolism present in the Tarot cards.

As I studied and learned more about (chi) energy from my husband and my instructors, I sensed even more connections in the Tarot's Major Arcana cards. The Tarot is the embodiment of the traditions and systems of mysticism in the Western world. The mystic ideology of the Western world connects more with me than Eastern mysticism does. This is why Tarot-Chi™ was developed.

There are 78 cards in a typical Tarot deck, but we will be working only with the 22 Major Arcana cards. These major cards are especially powerful in their imagery. That is why we will focus only on them in this exercise system.

For each major card, I created a series of physical movements or poses, based on the traditional archetypal imagery of that card. Even though most of the beautiful artwork changes with each Tarot deck, much of the modern meaning and symbolism associated with the cards stays the same from deck to deck.

The Fool card is the first major card in the deck, although it is usually given the number zero. It is followed by the other 21 major cards: The Magician, The Priestess, The Empress, The Emperor, The Priest, The Lovers, The Chariot, Justice, The Hermit, The Wheel of Fortune, Strength, The Hanged Man, Death, Temperance, The Devil, The Tower, The Star, The Moon, The Sun, Judgement, and The World or The Universe.

(Sometimes the Fool card is counted as the last of the major cards. Sometimes a few other cards are switched or renamed by the deck's creator, depending on their view of how it should be used. We will stick with 0-21, Fool to The World.)

As I learned and worked with the Major Arcana cards, I began seeing stories in the cards. In this book and throughout the exercises, I want you to think of the 22 cards as telling the huge, arcing story of life itself! Seen this way, the cards are a psychological tool that will take you on a journey of life through feminine and masculine energies, power and weakness, struggle and success, sacrifice and glory, life and death. The archetypal images will speak to you and tell you a story IF you will listen.

Some people are afraid to even take a look at the Tarot. They are definitely missing out on some great artwork. In the past, Tarot has been demonized by some religious people. But there is nothing evil here. And we are certainly using it in this exercise system in a positive way. It is a tool to help us grow and be stronger. As a medieval, pictorial system the Tarot shows you archetypes of humanity and human life. The recurrent symbols used in the Tarot show influences and experiences that we might face in life, from birth to death and everything in between.

This exercise system is not based on any specific Tarot deck; it is based on the ideas and concepts in the cards that are common to all decks. You do not even need a deck to learn the poses! All you need is to follow along in the book and practice. If you do have a deck, then that can make your exercise journey through the Tarot even more powerful and useful for you. As you learn the poses in my system, bring out your specific cards and use them to help you understand and feel the energy.

Before you get started learning the poses, I want you to know that I am not a medical doctor or a physical therapist. Please do not start this or any other exercise program without talking first to your physician. She will probably be thrilled that you want to exercise more. Just make sure there is not some underlying medical condition that will get worse with exercise. If you choose to learn and practice this exercise system, you do so at your own risk. I am not responsible for any harm you might experience by moving, stretching, bending, or breathing in any of the ways that I explain in this book.

The full exercise routine takes about 11 minutes from the first deep breath to the last salute to the 4 directions. There are 22 "Forms" in this exercise system. Forms are patterns of poses that are associated with each major card. There are around 50 poses in the 22 forms of this exercise system. And there are over 250 individual movements that make up the poses. Whew, that's a lot of gentle movement. On average, each card form has 2-3 poses.

For each card, we will include photos to show you how to create those poses. Read through the instructions in the book and study the pictures. Then try to recreate the pose. The diagrams will show the standing positions. Just modify them for sitting if you need.

There is a "home" position where the entire series of forms begins and ends. At the end of many of the forms, your hands will come back to the home position before flowing into the next series of poses for the next card. Home position starts with you standing with feet slightly parted, hands on your stomach at the belly button level. Make sure you have about 6 feet to either side and behind you. Breathe in deeply and slowly, hold it, and then slowly breathe out; repeat 2 more times.

As you learn this system, you will notice that we are moving slowly and stretching deeply. Our goal is to move and exercise every part of the body, literally from the head to the toes! This will increase flexibility and stamina. We recommend starting out with shallow stretches and slight bends, but you can definitely stretch and bend deeply if you are capable and want to.

As you are learning this system, it might feel as if you need to stop and start each form. That is okay! It is just a part of the learning process. Very quickly, you will find that all the poses flow together. The goal is to have each pose flow into the next in a slow and steady movement.

Most of the arm and foot work in this system is simple, but it takes some coordination of movements. (Just keep practicing and it will get easier.) When you step out, if you are moving forward, then you will put the heel down first, followed by the toes. When you reverse that pose, you will lift up the toes first and then the heel. If you are stepping back in the pose, then usually the toes go down first, followed by the heel. When you need more help with the poses and forms, we have a website (www.tarot-chi.com) and we are developing a YouTube channel with resources to help you.

Tarot-Chi ™ is part of my daily exercise. The benefits I have experienced amaze me. I am 54 years old, have had 3 serious car wrecks (none were my fault), have chronic illnesses, and yet, I am stronger physically and mentally than I have ever been.

Tarot-Chi ™ has helped me strengthen my core, heal my back pain, strengthen my knees, increase my stamina, extend my flexibility and improve my physical balance. Along the way, my spiritual and emotional life has improved, too. I have received a lot of benefit for just 11 minutes of exercise each day. I am excited to share this journey with you and hope you will be blessed with increased energy and vitality for the rest of your life. Ready? Welcome to TAROT-CHI ™

NOTE: If you would like to be a Certified Tarot-Chi ™ Instructor, then we would love to welcome you to our holistic family. This system is trademarked, so you will need our foundation's legal authorization. It is fun and easy to teach! You can create a second stream of income while helping others in your community.

The process to become a certified instructor involves live training sessions directly with us. We can do in-person training in some instances, or we can also do training via video conference. During that time, you will learn the process and theory behind Tarot-Chi ™ and once you demonstrate an understanding of the system, you will be certified. It is that easy! All training is live so that you can understand the nuances of the system. We are currently certifying instructors throughout the USA and beyond.

Once certified, our foundation will help and support you with marketing, further training, setting up a locale or area for classes, and ways to reach out to the community around you. Our goal is to encourage anyone and everyone that exercise is easy, fun and effective. We want classes to be open to everyone of all fitness levels, including those who are disabled, wheel-chair bound, and elderly.

We will certify only 1 instructor in an area, depending on the density of the locale and its ability to support your local small businesses. There are several options for class structure and payments. We will help you decide what is best for your situation and location. We will help you check the zip codes in your region that would be best for your new business venture. This way, you won't face competition from other Tarot-Chi ™ instructors.

Reach out to us on the website for more information. We look forward to hearing from you and welcoming you to our holistic family.

THE FOOL

Chapter 1

You might be able to fool some people some of the time, but you cannot fool your own soul.

THE FOOL is the infant, the beginning, the innocent, the inexperienced. Often shown as a blissful, young person carrying a bundle tied to a stick, head up, staring into the sky and missing the fact that he is about to fall off a cliff. Only the yipping dog at his feet is trying to warn him and prevent disaster. Or possibly, it is trying to push him off the cliff? Either way, the fool is not connected to what is around him, he is blissfully ignorant. But that is about to change!

We have all been that person about to make some major mistake or about to learn a major lesson. We have all had to begin again. Life is just a series of beginnings and endings, so we often have the chance to be the fool.

The series of poses for this card begins by stepping back with the right foot while lifting both arms to the side with the palms up.

Then bring your arms down and your foot back to home. Then the left foot goes back while the arms go up.

Do this series of poses twice on both sides, with the addition the second time of stepping back a bit further and tilting your head back as you raise your arms. If you are comfortable with your balance, you can lift the toes of your front foot up and get a good stretch in your foot.

That second time, put a big smile on your face! You will be feeling the spirit and energy of a new beginning, the spirit and energy of The Fool. In this set of poses, when you lift your arms, the goal is to move slowly and develop a deep, expansive stretch. You will come back to the Home position before transitioning into the next set of poses.

There is seldom a time in Tarot-Chi ™ where the movement just stops. The goal is to have slow, constant movement and muscle expansion. As we go through the poses, I will mention if there is a full stop and note where and why.

Physical Movement/Energy Focus:

Arms, Hips, Legs, Feet

GO A LITTLE DEEPER:

As you practice the movements of this card, see if you can mentally focus on and feel the difference when you add the head tilt and the smile during the second set of poses. Not only does a smile bring positive mental attitude to the position, but it reminds us to keep a light heart and a light perspective as we begin new adventures. At some point in life, we will be a fool. It is a part of the human condition. We will fail, and we will fail spectacularly. If it hasn't happened to you, then just know that it will at some point. The card reminds us that we humans all share this particular foible. So, keep negative judgements of yourself and others at bay.

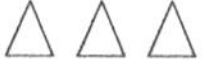

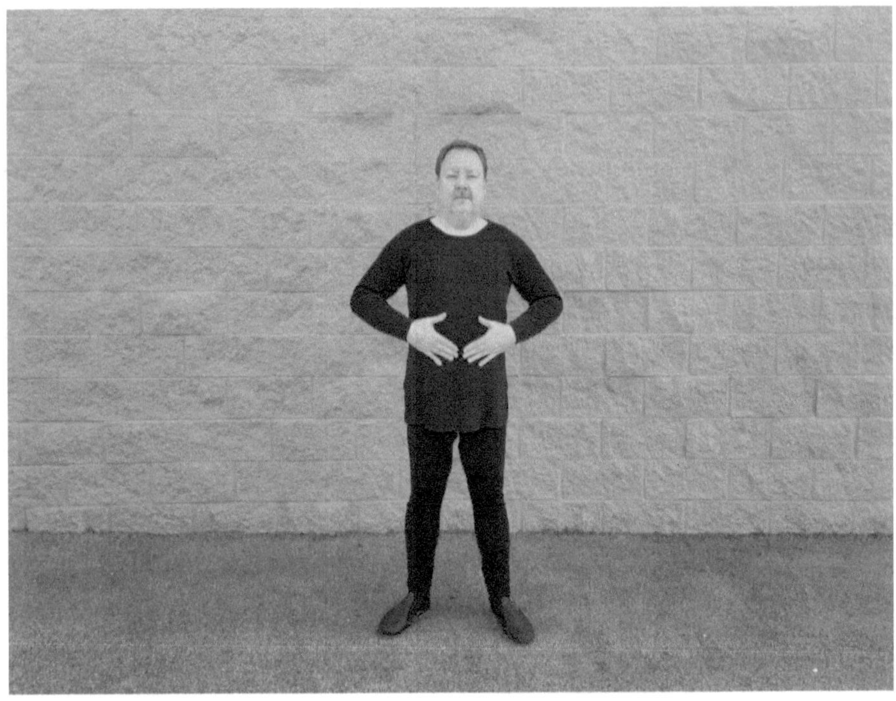

Figure 1 – Beginning Pose. This is also the End Pose. Take 3 deep breaths in through the nose and out through the mouth. Then we are ready to begin with our exercises.

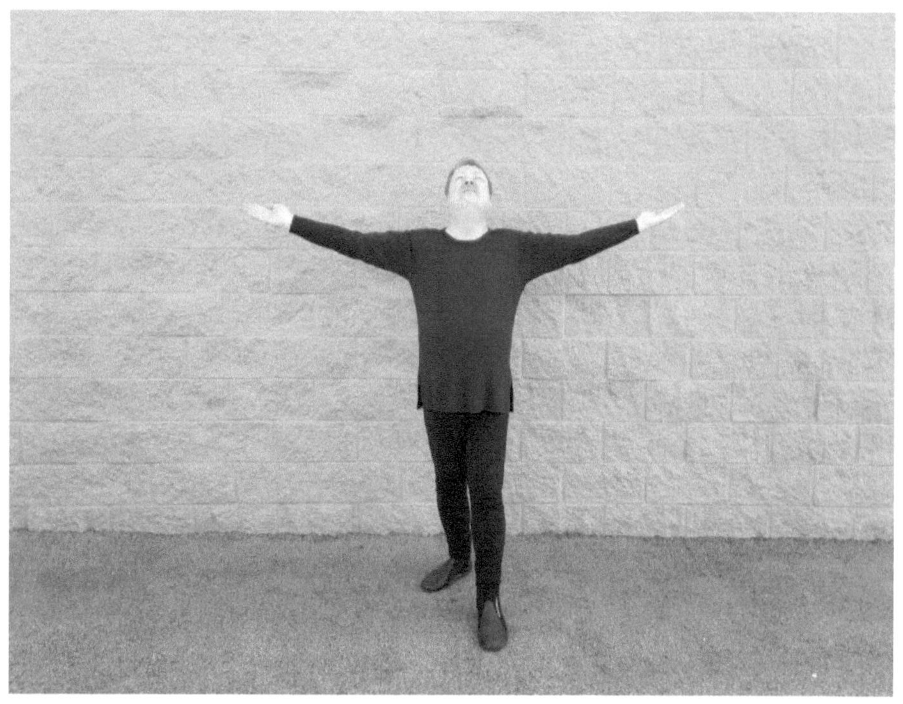

Figure 2 – You will step back, and raise your arms. Step forward and then repeat with the other foot.

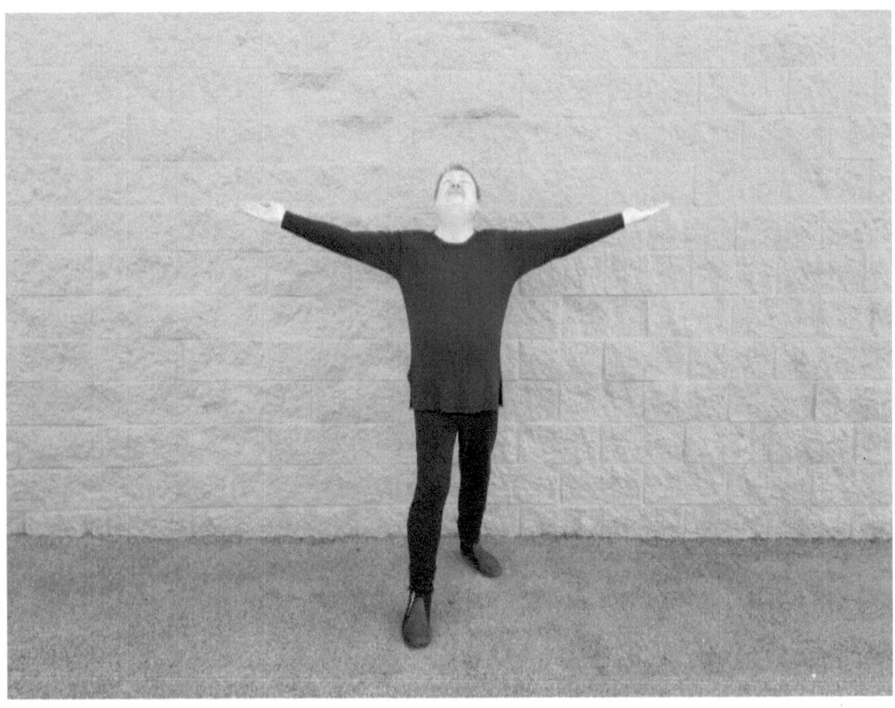

Figure 3 – When you step back for the second time, when you raise your arms, also tilt the head back and smile.

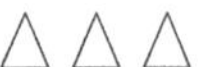

THE MAGICIAN

Chapter 2

What is "magic?" Stage magicians use props to perform tricks. Life magicians use tools to align their desires with natural forces.

THE MAGICIAN stands ready, his wand held in the air and his other hand pointing to the earth. Sometimes, this figure is shown as a juggler. Either way, the person has items on the table and items held in their hands. If he can balance all the items, then he is a master. (Life often feels like a juggling act, doesn't it?) If he can bring grace, virtue and light from heaven above to earth below, then he is a true magician, indeed. He is usually depicted standing behind a table where there are symbols of the 4 classical elements - earth, air, fire, and water.

The poses for this card will give us another deep stretch. First, your right hand goes up in the air at your side, holding your invisible wand. At the same time, you will look down at your left hand which is palm open, and pointing down to the ground. Then your hands come slowly back to center and you switch position, the left goes up and holds a wand while the right goes down, pointing to the floor.

Finally, you will do the same poses again, with a few additional stretches. As you get ready to lift your right arm into the air, you will lift your left knee up high and then step out to the left. When you point to the ground, you will stretch out the leg on that same side and point your toes. (Mark and I call this the disco dancing pose!) Then you will lift your left knee up as everything comes back to center. You do the same movements now with the right knee and the alternating hand positions.

With most of the stretches in this system, remember that the goal is slow and steady movement. There is also an opportunity for deep movements. Basically, you can extend most of these stretches into a very elongated pose. Or, you can keep the movement and poses simpler and shallower as needed.

Come back to the beginning home position at the end of each set of poses. Stand straight, with your feet slightly parted, your hands on your stomach at your belly button level.

Eventually, as you learn and practice, all the motions from the forms will flow together. For now, it is okay if it feels like you are starting and stopping for each card.

Movement/Energy Focus:

Arms, Hands, Hips, Shoulders, Neck, Feet, Toes

GO A LITTLE DEEPER:

As you practice this card, you can choose to vary the hand positions depending on your thoughts and needs at the time. With the hand that is held high, you can think of holding a wand, a candle, or even a sword. Mentally change the item you imagine holding high depending on what you are facing that day. If you are needing inspiration, think of a candle or a lantern held high in the darkness. If you are needing to do battle of some sort think of a wand or sword as the image of your intellect and your will charging into the fray.

With the hand that points down, you can also choose to hold the palm up or the palm down. Palm up is a more receptive position, like when you need inspiration. Palm down is a more active focused position where you are projecting your will and desires.

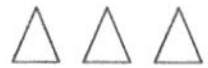

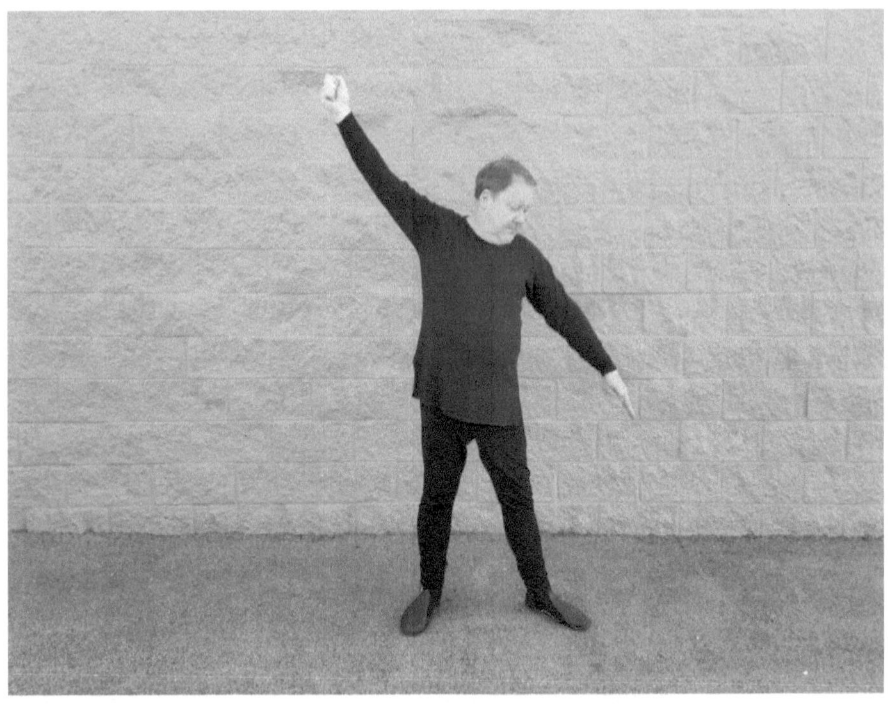

Figure 4 - As the Magician, you will hold a wand or candle aloft, and point to the ground with the other hand.

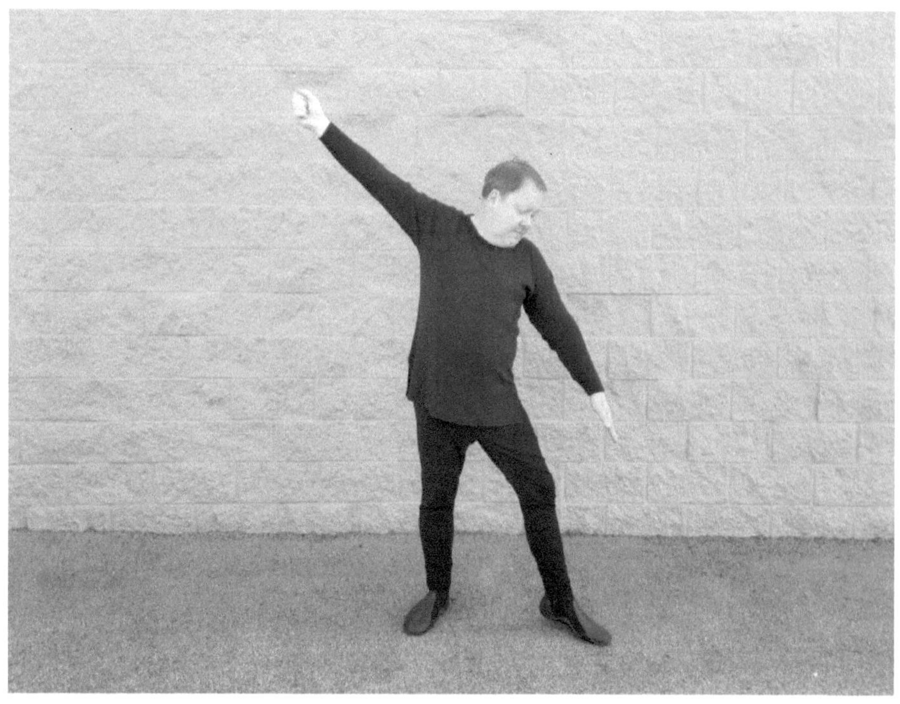

Figure 5 – This pose is the same as the prior pose, with the addition of pointing the toes. We call this the Disco Pose!

△△△

THE PRIESTESS

Chapter 3

True feminine power comes when you develop your inner emotional strength; it will allow you to face negatives in life and turn them into positives.

THE PRIESTESS has been associated with several feminine legends – the female Pope Joan, the Virgin Mary, Isis, Juno, Hera, and other powerful women from religious stories. As the embodiment of divine feminine power in human form, she invites you to come and commune with the ultimate feminine Divine. She is full of wisdom and knowledge. Often, she is shown holding a scroll or a book. Is it a book of wisdom? Is it a book of secrets?

We will be opening and closing a scroll in the poses for this card. First, our arms will go straight up, like two pillars in a temple. As your hands come back down, you will place your closed fists together in front of you, symbolizing the closed scroll.

We begin by turning the torso slightly to the left. You will take one step out with your left foot, placing your heel down first and then your toes. At the same time, you will rotate your hands until the left hand is on top of the closed scroll. And then you will open the scroll! The goal here is to have as deep of a stretch in your back, lower arm as possible. Get a really deep stretch on.

Those steps will be reversed back to the beginning position of the form, and you will make the same movements to the right. This time your right hand is on top of the scroll as you open it.

Do that entire series of movements, both to the left and then to the right, one more time, with one difference. You will not rotate your hands. This time, the scroll will be opened horizontally instead of vertically. Get a really good stretch in your arms, chest and back. Shift all your weight to the front leg, lifting your back heel.

Come back to the centered home position with your feet slightly parted and your open hands on your stomach at the level of your belly button.

<u>Movement/Energy Focus:</u>

Arms, Shoulders, Hands, Legs, Feet

<u>GO A LITTLE DEEPER:</u>

This is one of my favorite cards. The feminine leader, mystic or priestess has all too often been ignored in modern religions. I am so thankful for those religious organizations that encourage and welcome the feminine perspective as equal to the male. That is a refreshing turn back to the era when women were seen as capable of leading and capable of communing with the Divine.

As you open and close the scroll, think of whether you can live your life as an open book or open scroll. Can you be or become who you truly are? Humans are scared of the judgement from other humans, and with good reason. There is a lot of negativity and hate spread around the world. If you are fully free to live your life, are others able to live freely around you without judgement?

As you recognize the spark of humanity within every person, you will be able to live your life more as an open scroll or an open book. As you recognize the spark of divinity within every person, others will be able to live more openly around you.

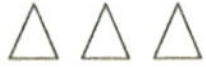

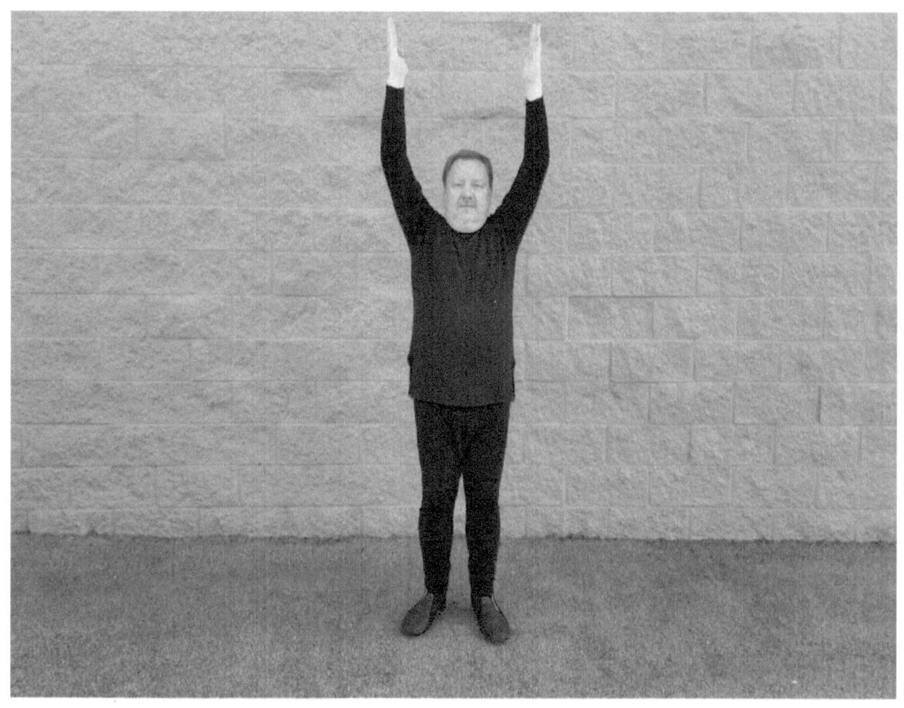

Figure 6 - This series begins by holding both arms straight up to signify two towers.

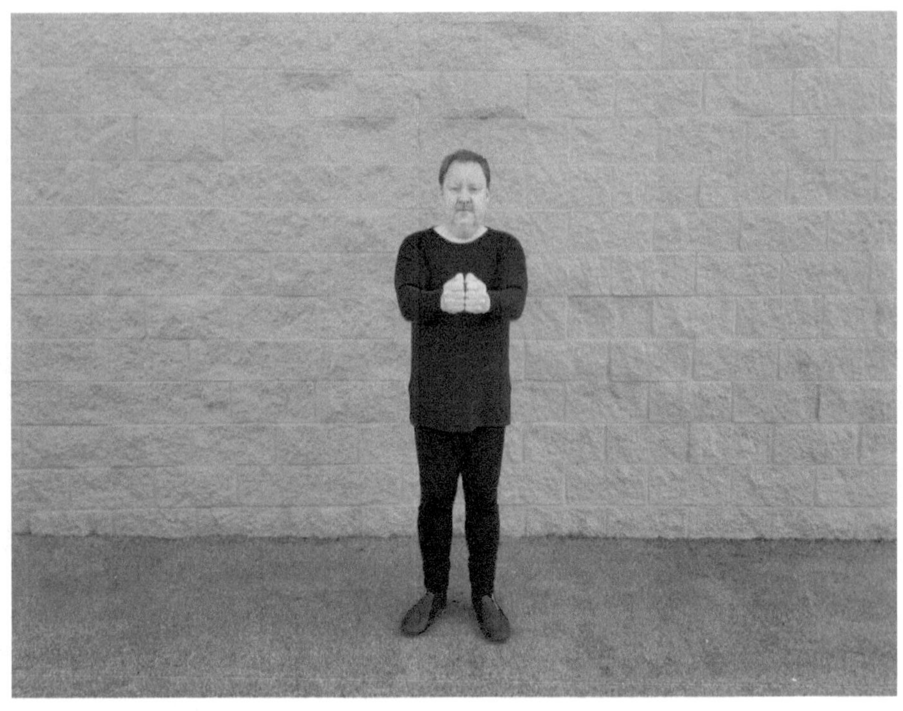

Figure 7 - Your fists come together in front of you. This is to signify a closed book or scroll of secrets.

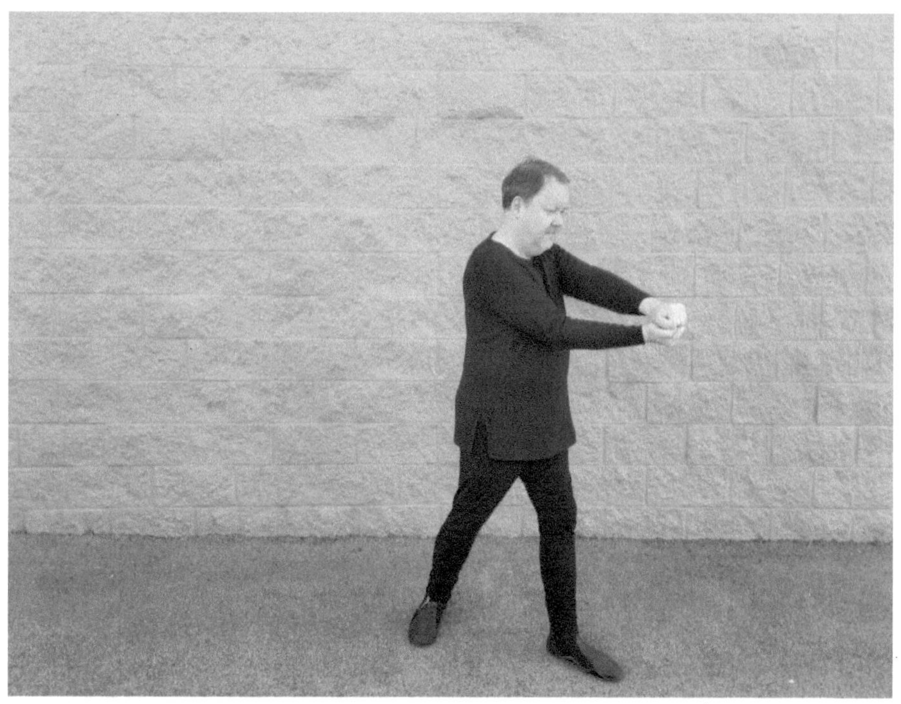

Figure 8 - Step to the left and get ready to open the scroll. You will open the scroll vertically, then step to the right and repeat the movement.

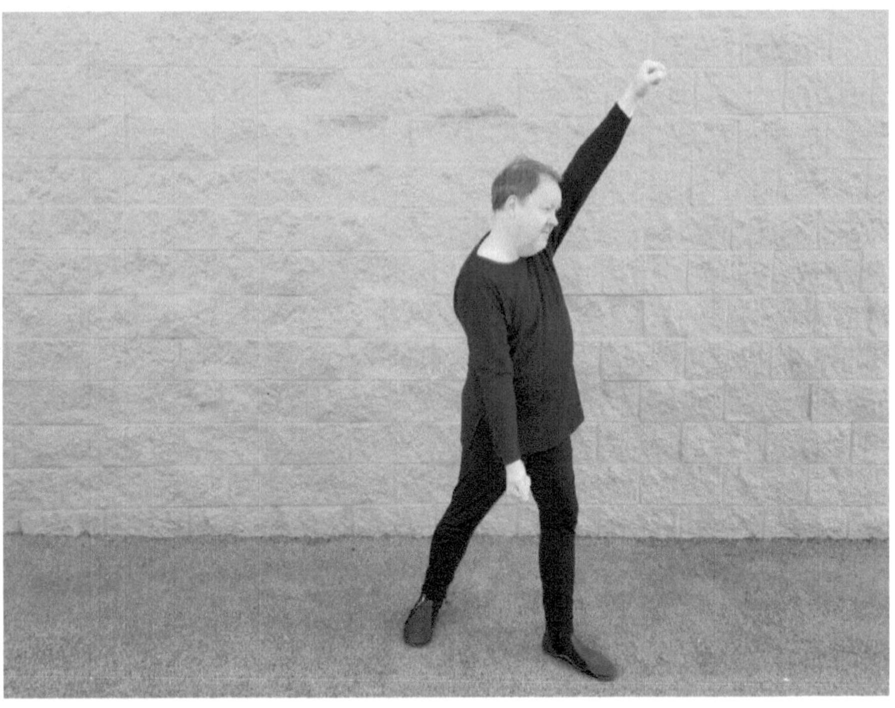

Figure 9 – The scroll has been opened. This movement will be repeated on the opposite side.

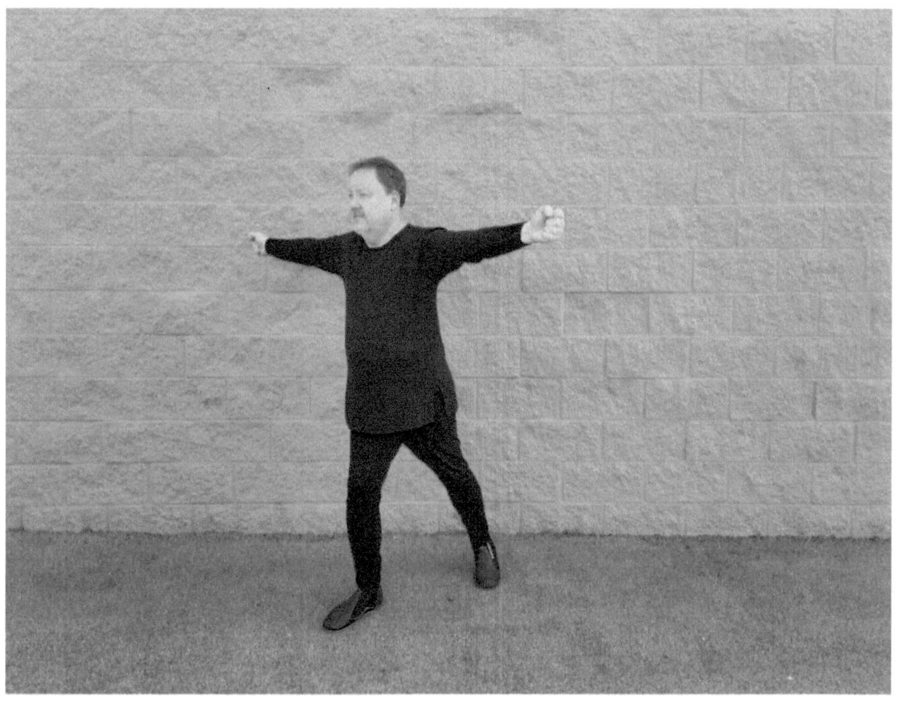

Figure 10 – Opening the scroll horizontally. After opening the scroll vertically, you will then repeat the foot movements while altering the arm movements.

△△△

THE EMPRESS

Chapter 4

Women have superpowers. We bring forth life and nurture it. We heal, we bless, we create. We are sisters, mothers, and lovers!

THE EMPRESS represents the power of birth and fertility. She is the gateway to human life. While the prior card was feminine power that leads to the Divine, this card is feminine power that leads to the divinely human. The Empress is a mother and creator, so she is often shown in the later stages of pregnancy. She is also often shown in a garden setting, with flowers and blossoming nature all around. It is a card of growth and possibility. In this way, the card is less about traditional gender roles and more about life-giving and life-nurturing sustenance. Masculine folks can get in touch with their feminine aspects, too.

We will be creating these poses by gathering up the nurturing, creative energy that is pulsing below your feet. The Earth is the true mother of us all. Without food, water and air from our planet, all life would die out.

From the home position, you will open your arms and bend down as if you are about to pick up a large ball, like the size of a beach ball. I want you to imagine this ball of energy, to really feel it pulsing and emanating from Mother Earth below your feet and then to really feel it between your hands. As you pick up the invisible ball of earth energy, imagine it there, feel it warming your hands and arms. You might find that your hands get hot. And you might find that other areas of your body also grow warm. Just know that you are connecting with and bringing earth energy into your body.

Bring the ball of energy up and hold it over your stomach and solar plexus area. Imagine healing energy flowing into your hips, thighs, groin and stomach. Now, bring the ball of energy up and into your lungs and heart area. Imagine healing energy flowing into you.

Finally, bring the ball of Earth energy up and over your head. Imagine healing energy now covering your entire body. If you are familiar with the Chakras and the colors associated with those energetic body centers, then you can imagine the colors of the rainbow as you bring the energy up and into your body.

Bend over and reach down for another "beach ball" of Mother Earth energy! Do the whole series of poses again, and end at the home pose.

Movement/Energy Focus:

Arms, Hands, Torso, Waist

GO A LITTLE DEEPER:

Modern physics teaches us that all life is energy. And all energy is moving bits or particles that are tiny and invisible. Try to imagine these tiny, vibrating bits of energy surrounding you. Now try to conceptualize that YOU are made up of that same energy, those same vibrations. We are truly children of the Universe.

When you first begin with this pose, since there is no fancy footwork involved, you can try it with eyes closed. As you bend over with eyes closed, imagine the energy of the Earth pulsing at your feet. As you pick up a ball of it, you just might be surprised that you can actually feel warmth in your hands and arms. You might think, ah, the power of my imagination. But really, it is the actual power of the Earth energy that surrounds us all. And now, you are more aware of it and focused on feeling it around and inside of you.

△△△

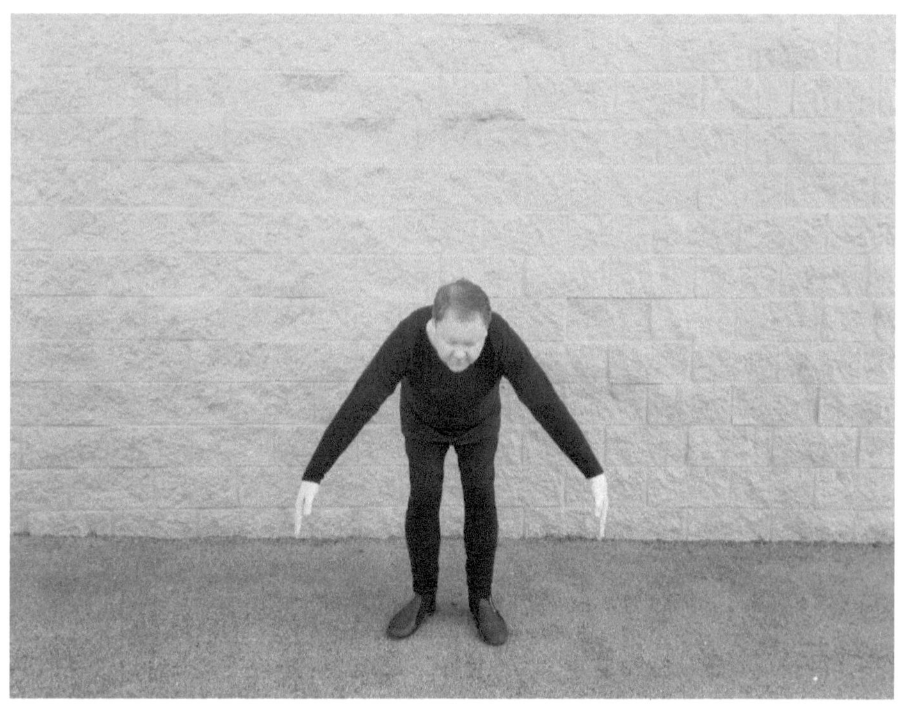

Figure 11 – Bending down to grab a ball of energy directly from the source, the Earth!

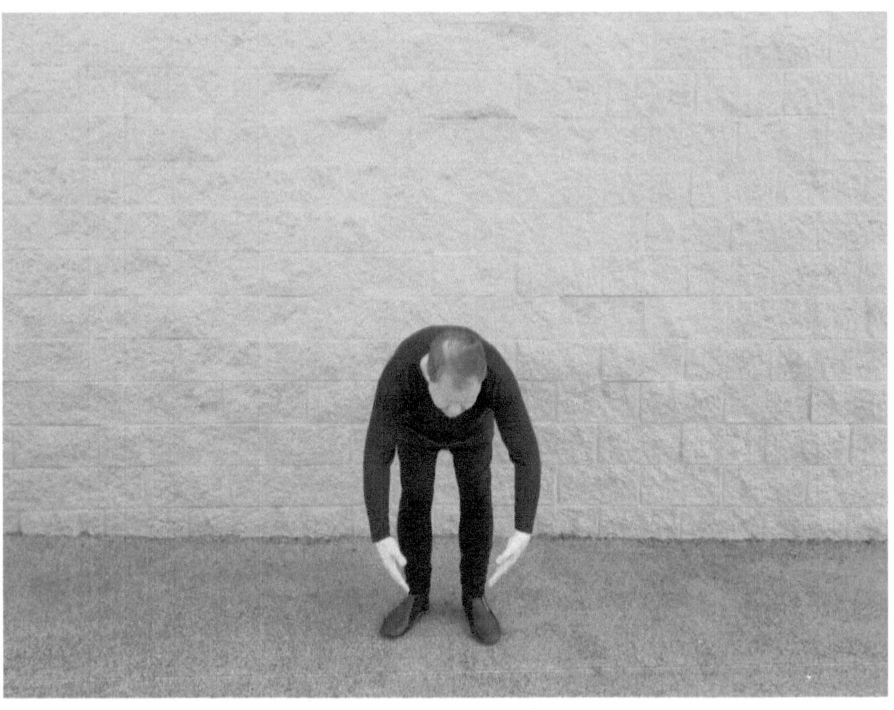

Figure 12 – Holding the ball of Earth energy. Imagine it as the size of a beach ball.

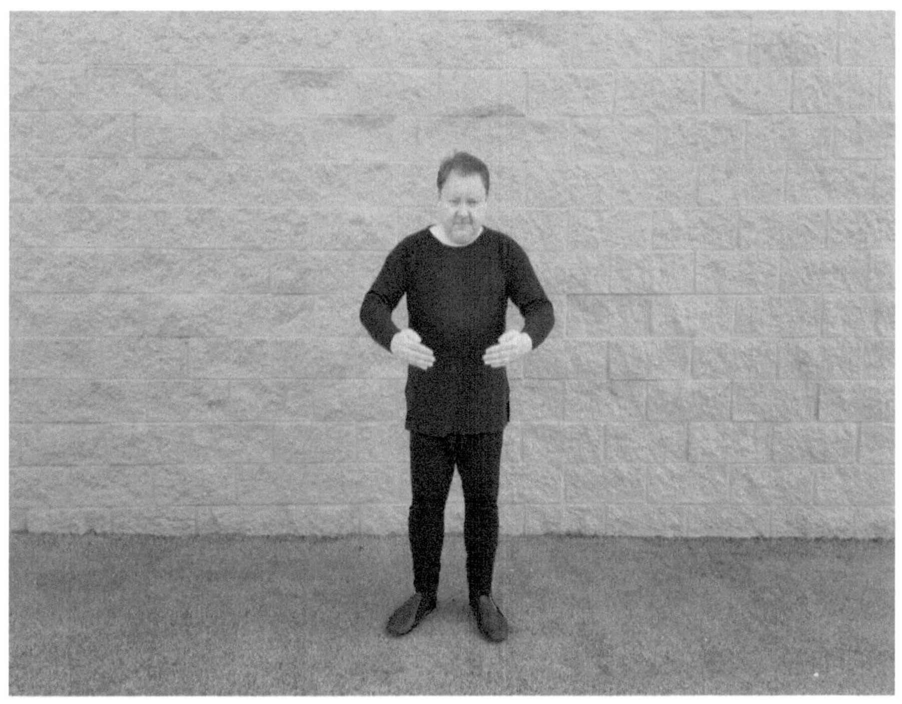

Figure 13 – Bringing the ball of energy up and into the body. First, over the groin and stomach area.

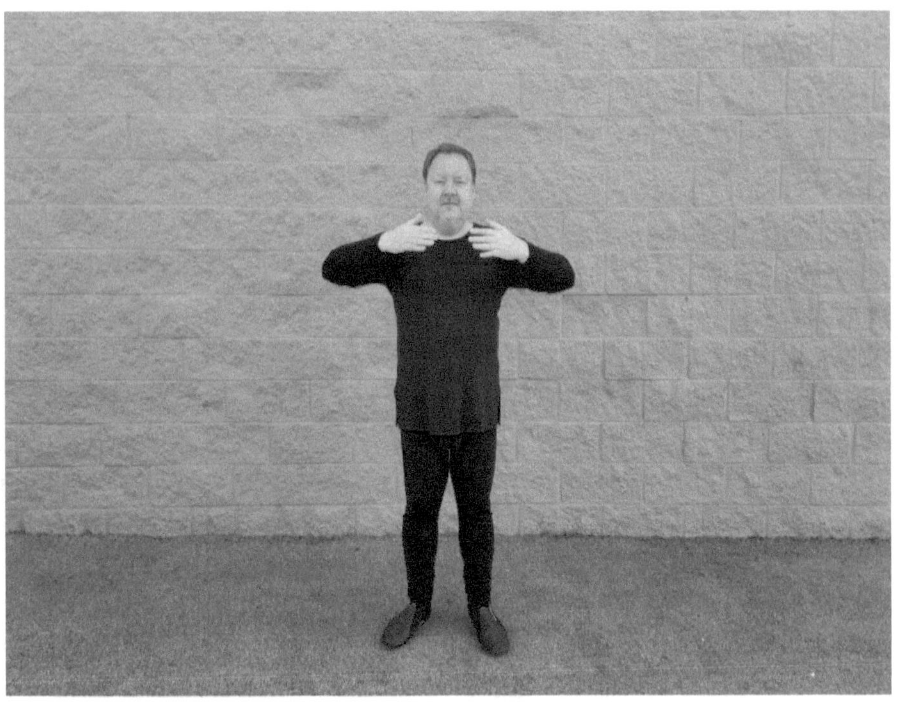

Figure 14 – Bringing the ball of energy up and into the body. Focusing on the heart and neck area.

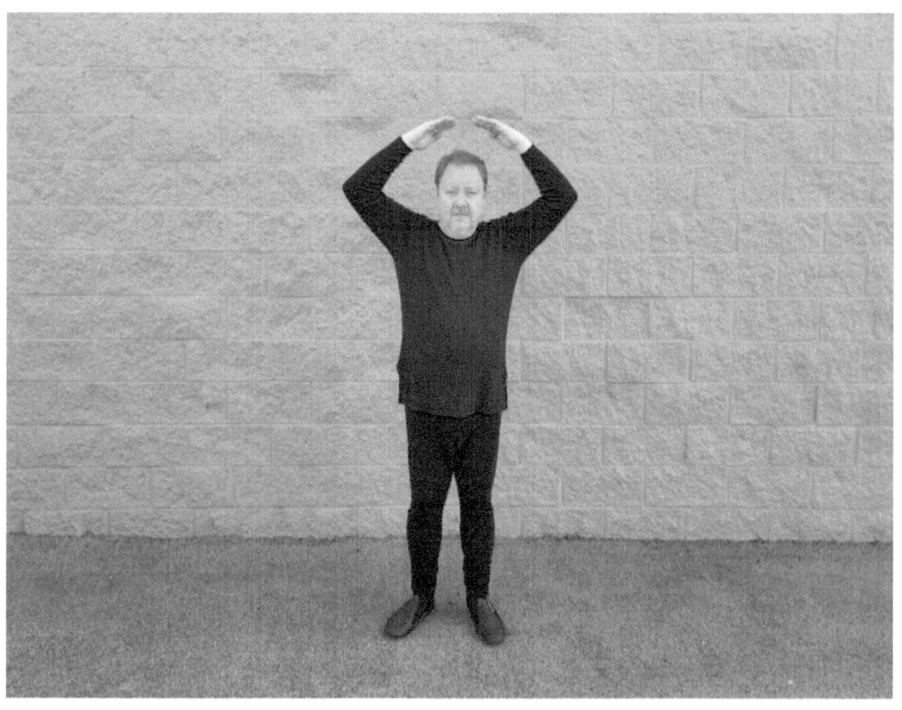

Figure 15 - The ball of energy will be brought up and over the torso area first, then also the heart area, and finally the head.

△△△

THE EMPEROR

Chapter 5

The ultimate masculine energy is penetrating, strong, direct, full of vitality and energy; and yet tender enough to hold and protect a new-born.

THE EMPEROR is the absolute ruler of his world. He is all about stability and power, and as the ruler, his word is law. This is also about the penetrating capabilities of man. I am not just talking about sexuality, but also about intellectual and psychological penetration. The forceful use of a person's skills to bless, heal, or even save another is a penetrating use of force. The energy here is not about power used against someone's will, that sort of use of power is negative and about domination. This energy is about power, but used with ultimate control.

For this series of poses, we will be squatting down as if sitting on a throne. Get ready for your thighs to burn a bit, because the deeper your squat, the more intense the feeling. You will maintain the squat during this entire form.

Your hands are firmly clenched at waist-height in front of you, as if holding double sceptres or staffs. The energy of this card is directly focused, looking neither to the left or right. But we will be taking time to get in a good neck stretch, turning your head slowly and fully to look to the left, and then slowly and fully to the right. Maintain the squat the whole time.

My husband suggested this next movement as an indication of penetrating force. As you are squatting down, with your hands firmly held in front of you, slowly extend first one arm and then the other, as if you are holding forth your staff, the symbol of your power. Display your staff with your arm fully extended, taking alternating turns twice for each arm. Stand up out of the squat, and return to the home position. Do you feel the burn?

<u>Movement/Energy Focus:</u>
Arms, Neck, Hands, Thighs, Knees

<u>GO A LITTLE DEEPER:</u>

With most of the forms or poses, you have the option to expend a little more physical energy and stretch deeper. You have that opportunity with this card during the squat. I have some knee damage due to car wrecks, so I am not able to deeply bend with the knees, but you might be able to.

There is also a chance for a deeper stretch in the arm extension. When you extend one arm out fully, you can also pull back with the other arm. Instead of looking like you are holding forth a staff, this will look more like the pose of an archer, which is a very masculine and penetrating pose, also.

With many of the cards in the Tarot, there might be traditional gender associations – a man on this card, a woman on the previous. But these cards do not have to be about specific genders; think of them instead as being about personality aspects that we all have inside us. Maybe you need to feel a little more of the firey boss-man aspect of this card, or more of the nurturing, calm aspect of another. So, think of the cards not as gender-specific, but as the human aspects that we all have inside. This is the duality, or plurality, of human nature. We have many parts of our personalities on display at any time. Some parts may need to be strengthened for a specific task or problem, so let the cards guide you or speak to you. If you feel drawn to a certain card or movement, then focus on why you feel that way and spend some time in contemplation.

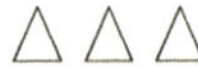

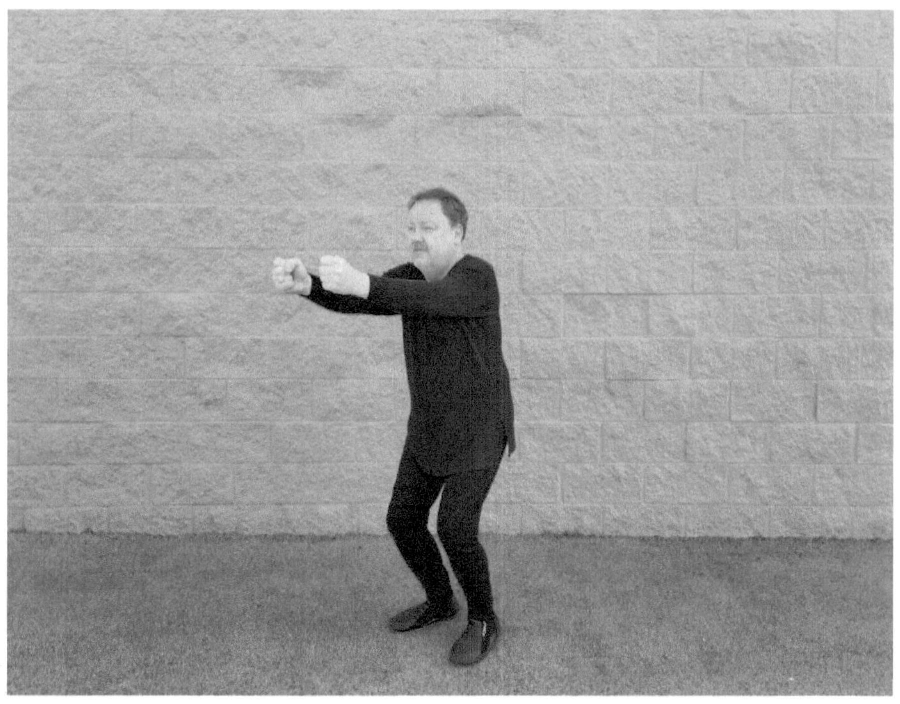

Figure 16 – The Emperor squat. From this position, we will take a moment to get in a few neck stretches before the thrusting stretches.

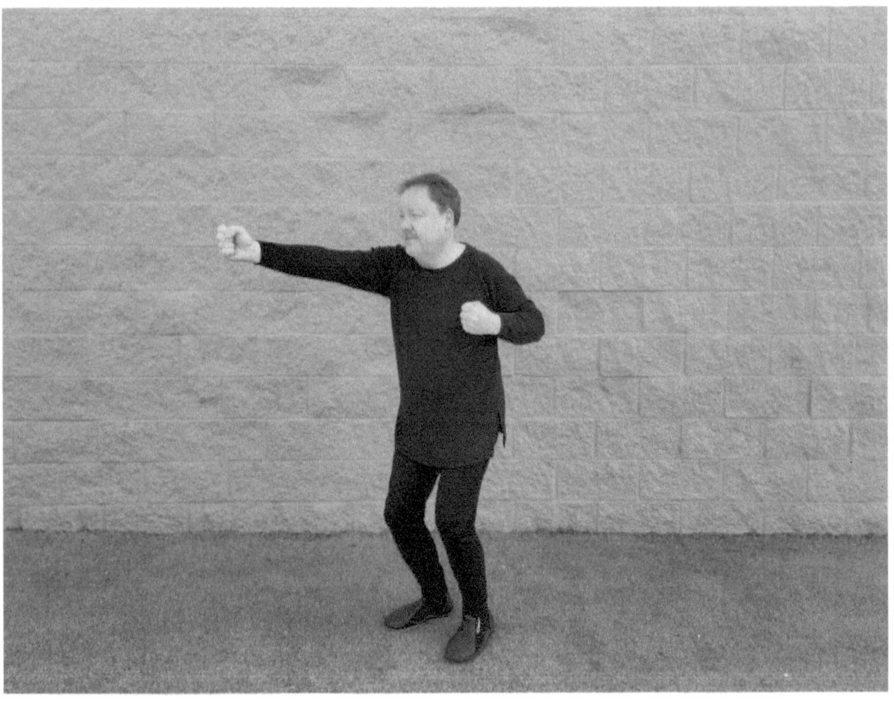

Figure 17 – From the deep squat, the arms are extended twice each, alternating, in a show of masculine power and authority. Imagine holding out a staff or sword.

△ △ △

THE PRIEST

Chapter 6

Your connection to the Divine belongs to you! No religious leader can come between that relationship. And none should try.

THE PRIEST and the Priestess are often seen as complimentary cards, with male and female religious energies pictured. This card is a typically masculine representation of a religious ruler. He is usually shown with a right hand lifted up delivering a blessing to the people that are clustered around. Often, two fingers point to the sky, and two fingers point to the earth, symbolizing the interface where heaven and earth come together. The religious leader (male or female) literally stands as a conduit to channel the energy from heaven to the earth. The Priest's goal is that as it is above, so shall it be below. He (or she) is literally bringing heaven to earth.

We are going to lift both arms up and point to the sky. Stretch fully, and then slowly bend over at the waist (flexing your knees as needed) to "bless the supplicants." Slowly rise up and then repeat the pose.

Remember that the Priest is making a gesture with his hands. You can make any hand gesture during this series of poses that you want. I would just recommend that you keep it positive! I always make the American Sign Language (ASL) sign for "I Love You." If you have a specific symbol or gesture that has meaning for you, then make or draw that symbol in the air as you stretch up. Whatever gesture holds meaning for you is the right one to use. And then come back to the home position after doing this pose twice.

<u>Movement/Energy Focus:</u>

Arms, Shoulders, Hands, Waist, Torso

<u>GO A LITTLE DEEPER:</u>

The blend of masculine and feminine aspects that you will see in the Tarot cards is similar to the duality of yin/yang in Oriental thought. Western ideology has not been quite as open and accepting of the dualities of light-dark, push-pull, male-female; but I think we are slowly getting there. The Priest/Priestess duality is similar to the Emperor/Empress duality. Both are necessary balances of the energies, one divine and the other divinely human.

If you want a deeper stretch with this form, then I recommend that you come up on your toes as you lift your arms skyward. Then lower your feet before you bend over in the Priest's benediction/blessing.

As an alternate, you can stand in a very Egyptian religious pose. Just take one step forward with your left foot. Keep both feet flat on the ground while you stretch up. You will look very much like a museum statue of Anubis or Osiris.

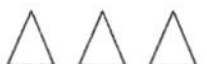

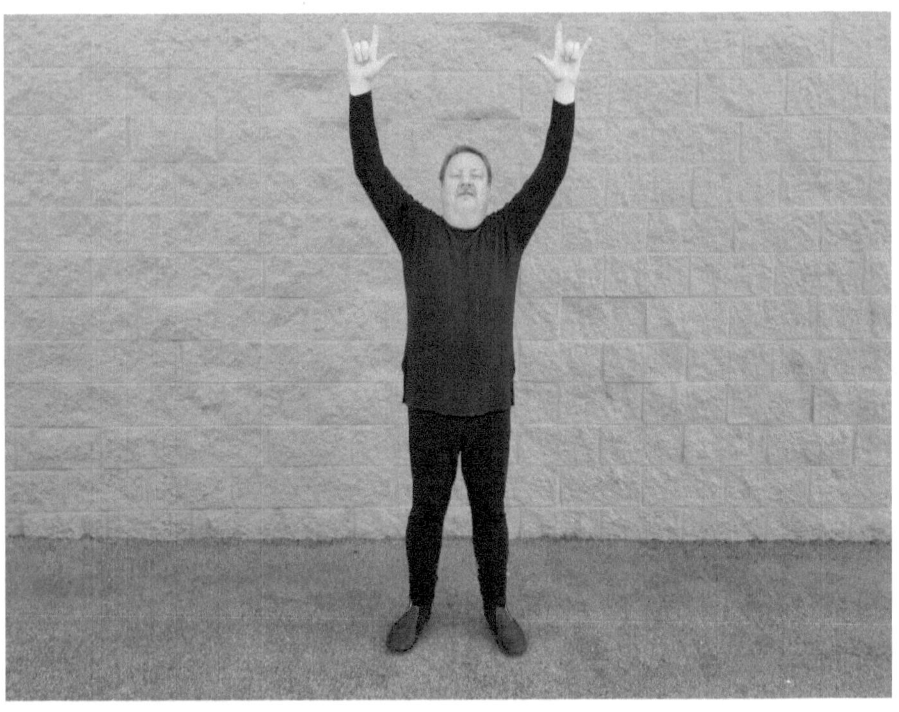

Figure 18 - Reach up to the sky and BE the physical connection between Heaven and Earth.

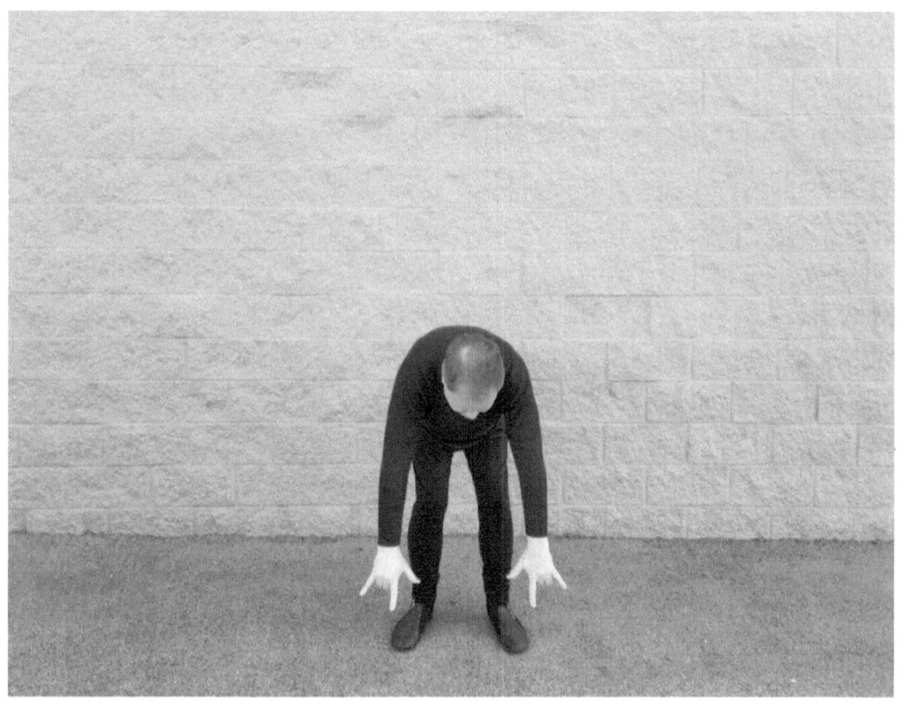

Figure 19 - We lean down to "Bless the Supplicants." I always use the American Sign Language symbol for "I love you" but use any (POSITIVE) symbol you choose.

△△△

THE LOVERS

Chapter 7

Male and female are too often seen as opposites, as two sides of some great divided dualism. But that is an illusion. The two natures are complementary and coexisting.

THE LOVERS are all about attraction, beauty, and irresistible forces. This card shows two coming together to make one power couple or a completely powerful force. This card is about relationships and choices. The imagery usually, almost always includes two naked figures, often pictured in a Garden of Eden setting. Of course, if it is the symbolic garden, then there is usually a serpent, too. Beware of the snakes!

In order to feel the energy of this card, we will be making several pivots and turns with our feet, while adding in some squats and hand gestures. First take a small step back with your right foot, toe first, while at the same time pivoting on your left heel. Both feet are now flat on the floor and you have made a quarter turn to the right. At the same time, you will make a shallow or deep squat, depending on your comfort level. As you bend and squat, extend your arms with the palms up, and beckon twice with both arms in a "come to me" sort of gesture. You will make four pivots with the squats and the arm/hand gestures, each time facing a new direction until you make it back to your beginning position.

As you do this movement, think of your lover, your partner, and all the wonderful moments that you share together and the blessings to come. I often think of the good things that we have planned, a trip, a visit with family, etc.

If you want one, but don't have a partner, then this is the perfect time to think of the attributes you desire in a life partner. Imagine your true love is standing across the room from you. Mentally (and physically) beckon to them. Call out to this imaginary partner, and invite them to come to you. Hey, you never know what kind of good things will come your way because of this card! Put out all the love you can into the world, and love will come back to you. And then come back to the home position.

<u>Movement/Energy Focus:</u>

Thighs, Feet, Arms, Hands

<u>GO A LITTLE DEEPER:</u>

I cannot stress enough how much putting out good vibes into the world will bring good vibes back to you. When you can take an awful situation and turn it to good by the sheer force of your intent and your will, then you have some seriously powerful skills. You want to attract love? Then BE love. You want a true lover and partner? Then BE a true and loving person. Be what you want to attract.

As I am doing all of these poses, I have little snippets of poetry rummaging around in my head. (Go read some Rumi love poetry if you need inspiration.) If you need love in your life, if you are looking for a lover, a partner, then put ALL of your good energy into this pose and this card. Send out as many good vibes as you can.

Get specific with the Universe. Make a list of the attributes you want in a partner. And ask for it. But be real. Real people are not perfect. Do not ask for perfection, because no one is perfect. Ask for real. Ask for love. Ask for heart and soul. And it will come to you!

△△△

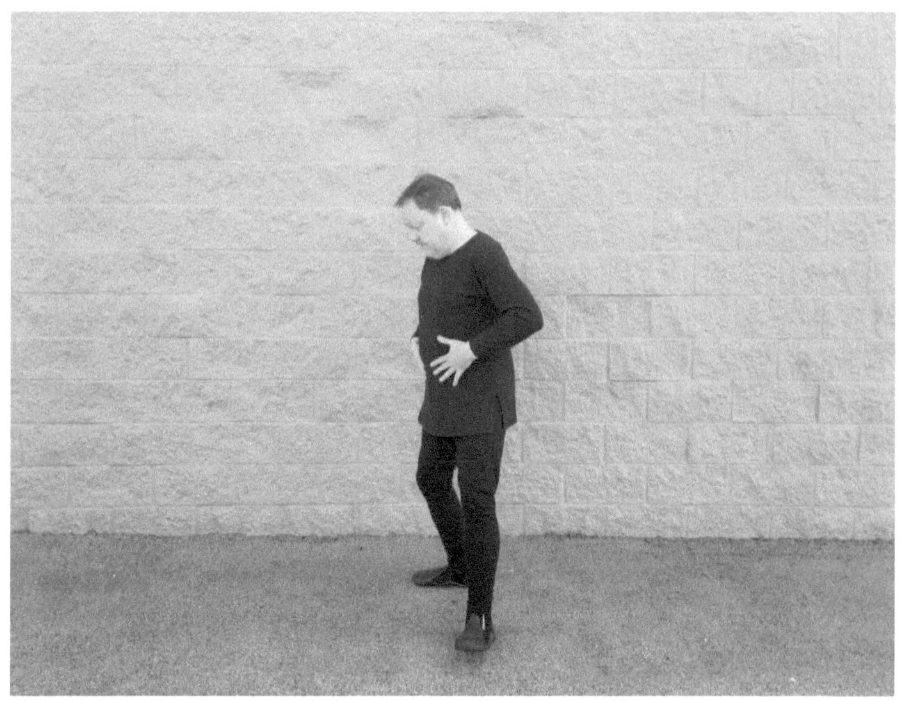

Figure 20- This pose has some fancy footwork that you will have to practice. As you step back and to the right, you pivot on the left heel.

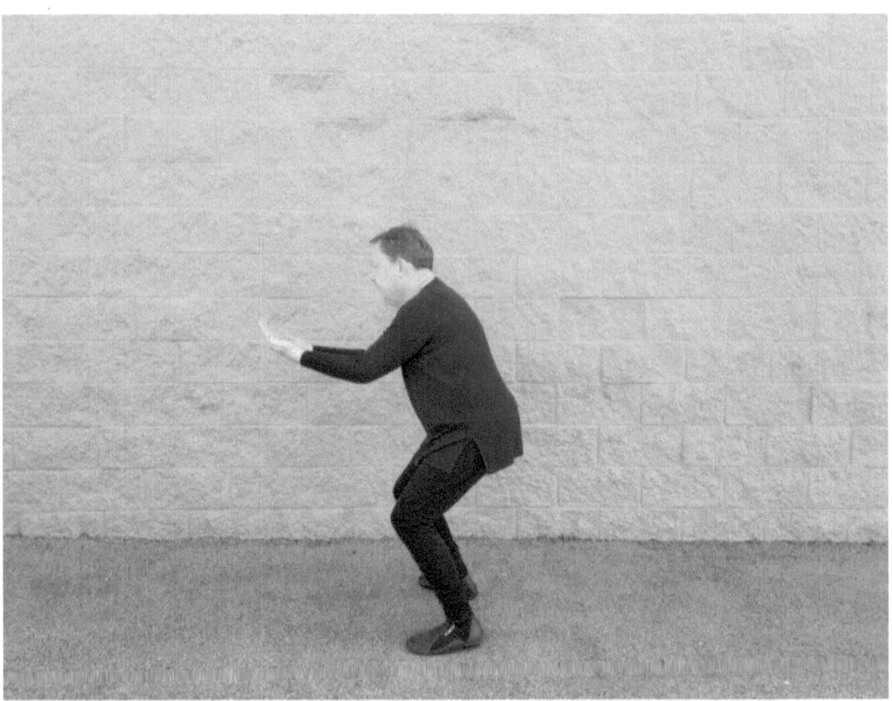

Figure 21 - After each pivot and turn, you will squat down and extend your arms while you beckon love to come to you.

△△△

THE CHARIOT

Chapter 8

You've just got to keep on rollin' – wherever the road takes you. OR chart your path instead and take control of the wheels.

THE CHARIOT is being pulled by animals, usually two horses, but sometimes more. At times, the chariot is pulled by mystical creatures. It depends on the artist and the theme of the card deck you have. But usually, there are creatures pulling a wheeled conveyance, and there is an enigmatic figure sitting inside. There is a definite feeling and indication of motion! The figure may be geared up for war, with helmet, chainmail and sword. The figure may look like it is off to battle. Or possibly, it is just going out to deliver messages.

Has the motion just stopped? Or is the motion just about to begin? The figure must keep the animals/creatures who are drawing the chariot or cart in line. Control of the forces must be maintained or oops, the conveyance might turn over.

We will focus on the large chariot wheels in motion. For this series of poses, you will begin by making large circular motions with your arms directly in front of you, rotating your hands around each other, pretending that your hands and arms are the wheels of that chariot.

Now, slightly lean back as the wheels climb higher and higher. Then slowly lean forward and down as the chariot wheels touch the earth. Bend your knees as needed. Come back up to the center. Now, keeping the wheels in motion, lean and twist to the right and then to the left. Come back to center again. Do this up and down, and then side to side motion twice before finally coming back to end at the home position.

<u>Movement/Energy Focus:</u>

Arms, Hands, Torso, Waist

<u>GO A LITTLE DEEPER:</u>

As the wheels climb higher and higher, you can lean back as far as you are comfortable. You can get a great stretch in your lower back this way. Just be careful of your neck. You do not want to over stretch your neck and you do not want to hold it in a stiff and uncomfortable position. If at any time you start to feel pain or discomfort, then stop that movement and speak with a professional doctor. Our goal is always to stretch and gain flexibility, but we do not want to cause damage or pain. When you stretch backwards, just go very slowly and be mindful of how your body is feeling and responding to the stretches.

The energy of this card is more about the choices you take for activity and action. You are the charioteer and in charge of the ride. How fast you go and if you stray from the path is all due to your attention or lack of. Use this time to think of the path you are on and whether you need to change direction.

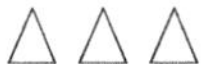

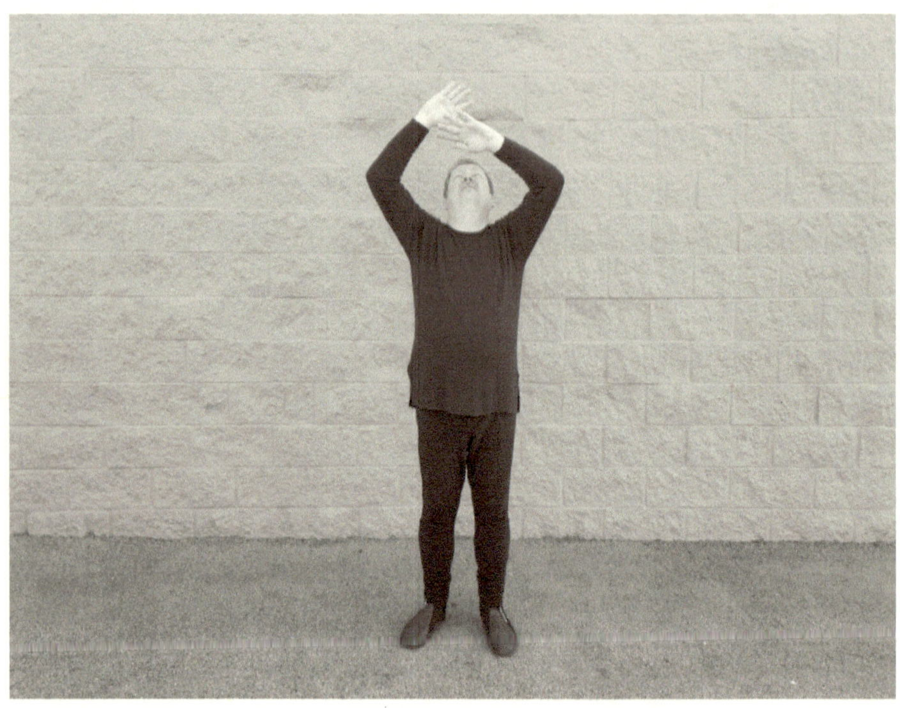

Figure 22 – Your hands circle around and around. You lean back and then lean all the way forward to show the wheels moving.

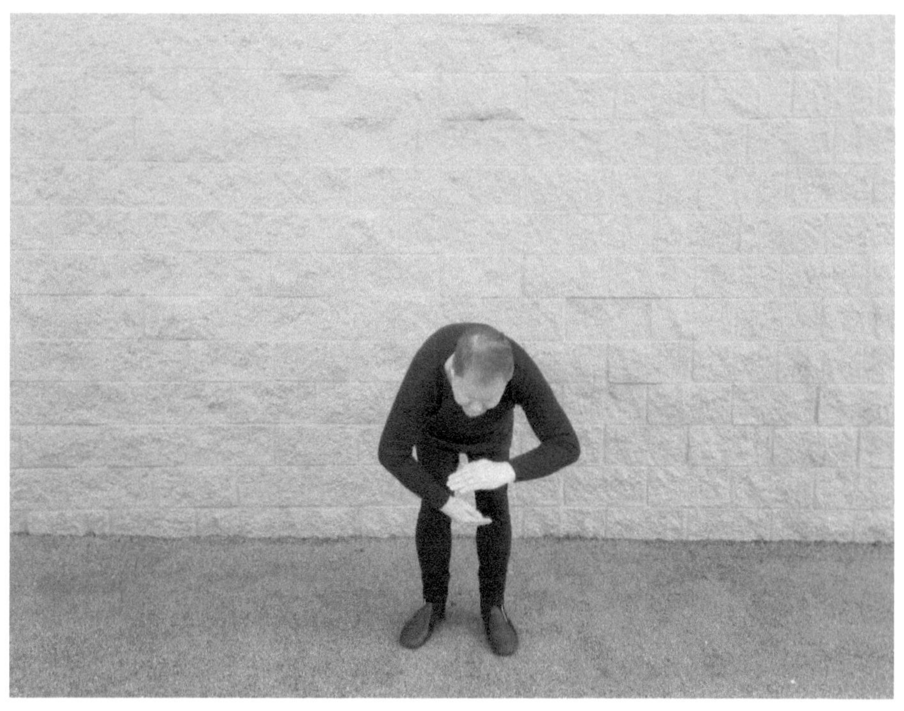

Figure 23 – The wheels of the Chariot moving down to the ground.

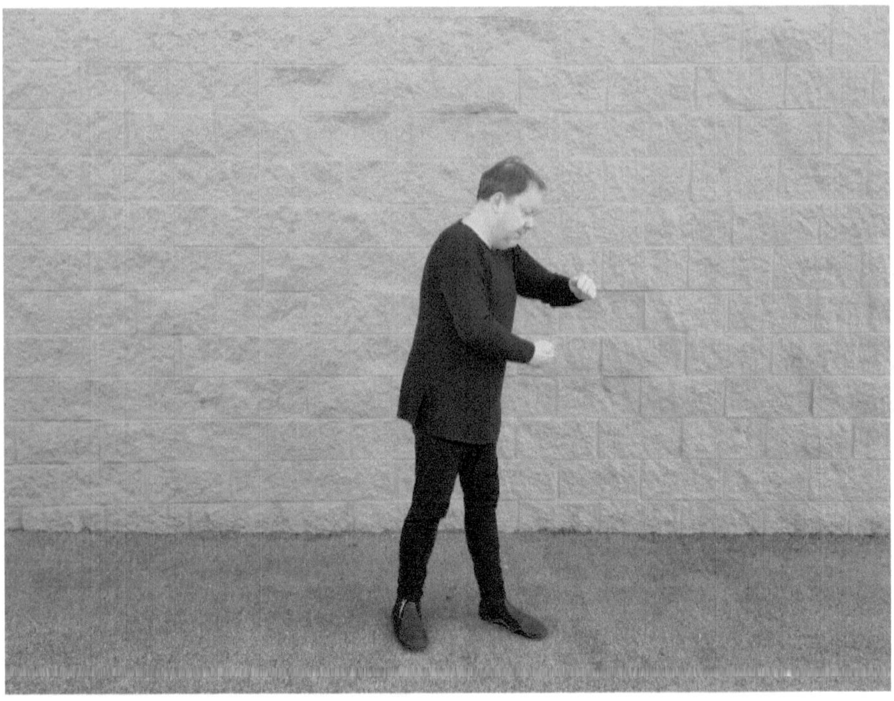

Figure 24 – Your hands, as the wheels of the Chariot, will move to the left and the right. Then you will repeat the entire series of moves again –up and down, right and left.

△△△

JUSTICE

Chapter 9

The nature of the law of Karma is not about retribution, it is about equilibrium. Nature is continually working to restore the balance that we keep disturbing.

JUSTICE – the law, right versus wrong, the judge, the jury, the verdict. And yet? The idea of Justice in Tarot is more than just about the workings of the human legal system. It is about the workings of the *universal* justice system. It is a balancing system that is impersonal and blind. It is the idea of Karma - that every action has a consequence, and that balance will be maintained by the natural forces at work in the Universe on every level.

The figure on the card often holds a scale, usually made of gold or some precious metal. Sometimes the figure is wearing a mask, showing that the balance of justice, of karma, is blind. It is equally given to all, without preference.

We will feel the energy of this card by using our hands as the representation of the scales. Extend your arms. Bring your hands out in front of you, palm up. Now, extend your arms to the side and prepare to swing them up and down, four times, alternating first right and then left, suggesting a scale. Bend at the waist as you swing your arms.

Now the movement changes slightly as you turn your upper torso 45 degrees to the left. You will once again swing your arms up and down, four times, alternating first right and then left. (You definitely can feel the stretch in your side and back as you do this.) Bring your upper torso back to the front. Now turn 45 degrees to the right and swing your arms up and down four times again, alternating right and left. You can definitely feel the stretch in your waist/torso muscles.

Movement/Energy Focus:

Arms, Shoulders, Torso, Waist

GO A LITTLE DEEPER:

You can make the bending movement at the waist as deep or as shallow as you choose. Deep stretches like these can be great at increasing flexibility. Just don't overstretch. Take it easy at first and then lengthen that stretch when you can.

When you think of the scales of justice, remember that we all have made mistakes. Do not stand in judgement of others, because you do not ever know what their path has been. You cannot look at someone and know the pain they carry around inside, so just be kind. Of course, be kind to yourself, too. The balance of the scales in life moves back and forth. Where one day, things are rough, another day they will be better. Use the time with this set of stretches to remind yourself that life has ups and downs - the goal is to be kind, loving and real through all of it.

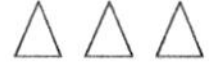

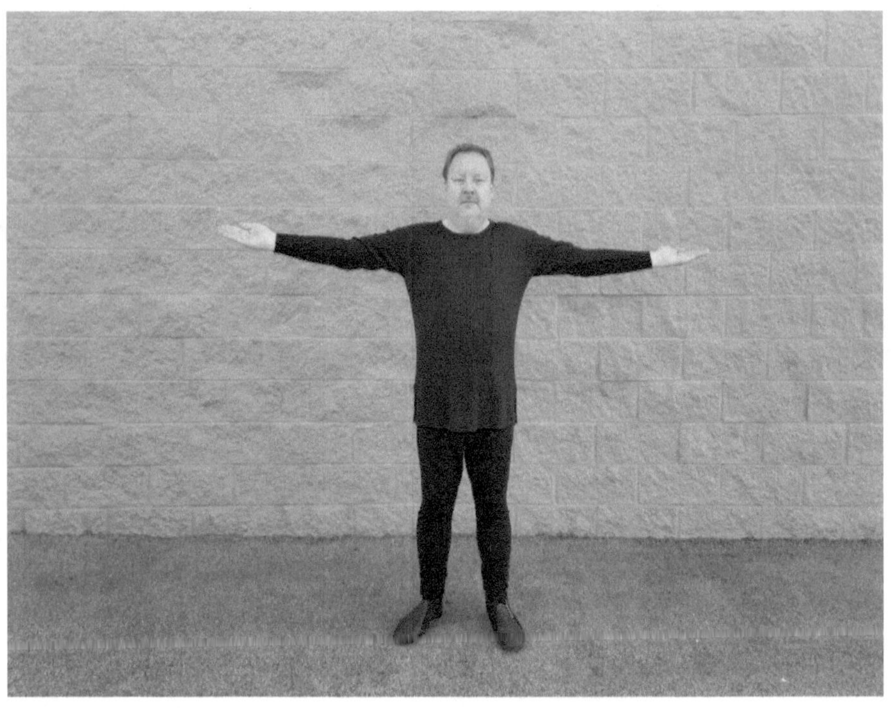

Figure 25 – We begin this series of poses by extending both arms directly out to the side.

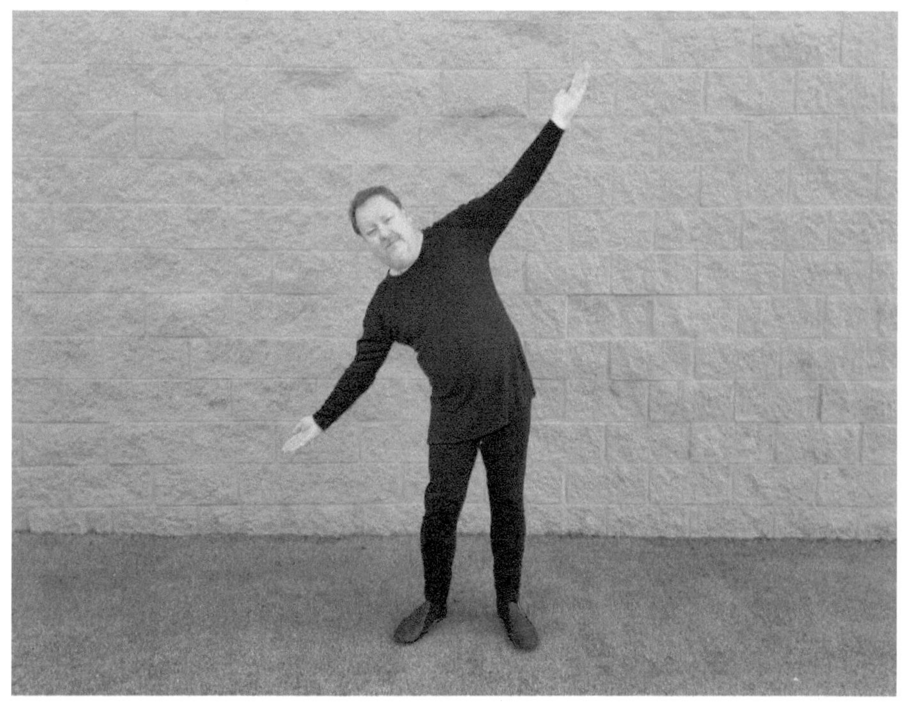

Figure 26 – Bend at the waist, first to the right and then the left. Do this two times.

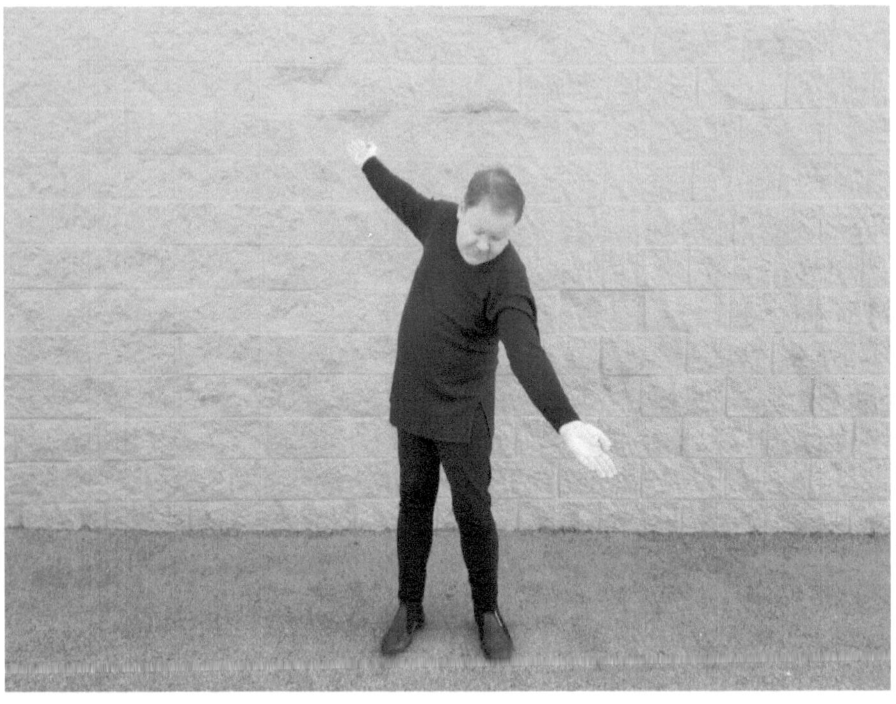

Figure 27 – Twist the upper torso a quarter-turn to the left. Bend at the waist again, first to the front and then the back, two times each.

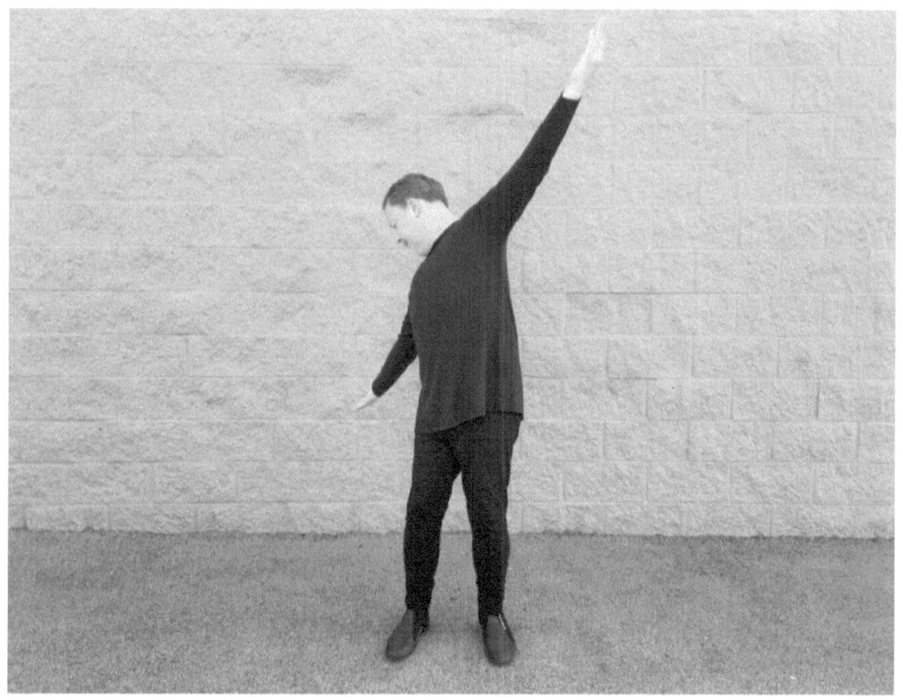

Figure 28 - Twist the upper torso a quarter-turn to the right. Bend at the waist again, first to the front and then the back, two times each.

△△△

THE HERMIT

Chapter 10

Today I will be a hermit. I will turn away from the world and all distractions. I will turn my focus instead to inner peace and growth.

THE HERMIT might just walk away and leave all his troubles behind. Would you like to be a hermit? Often, we will see a hooded figure standing alone in a desolate place, with a walking staff in one hand and a lantern in the other. Instead of walking away from our problems, we will use this card to gently shine the light of truth on our issues as we seek knowledge and enlightenment.

We are going to focus on long, slow, steady movements. Begin by bringing your right arm straight out and imagine holding a lantern in front of you. At the same time, your left arm comes in close to your shoulder to grasp a staff or walking stick.

We will slowly turn at the waist, a quarter-turn to the right, and then slowly back to the front. Turn again, slowly to the right, just a bit further, and slowly come back. On the third turn, you will step back with your right foot, as you slowly swing the lantern all the way back as far as you can, to look behind you. Slowly return to the front.

Repeat all the movements on the left side, first switching lantern and staff. As you do these movements, think of the resistance you feel when swinging your arms underwater – that is the slow, steady feeling I want you to create as you move your lantern. All the motions you make in Tarot-Chi ™ will be slow and steady. The goal is to have consistent and flowing movement at all times. And then you will go back to the home position.

Movement/Energy Focus:

Torso, Hands, Arms, Legs, Feet

GO A LITTLE DEEPER:

Every series of poses for each card in Tarot-chi can have a deeper meaning for you. Here, the lantern, the light of knowledge, is swung further and further back behind you.

Can you shine a light on your past? Can you bring any painful or negative deeds (those done TO you or those done BY you) into the light of today? Shining a bright positive, loving light on the past can be a powerful way to find forgiveness for yourself and for others.

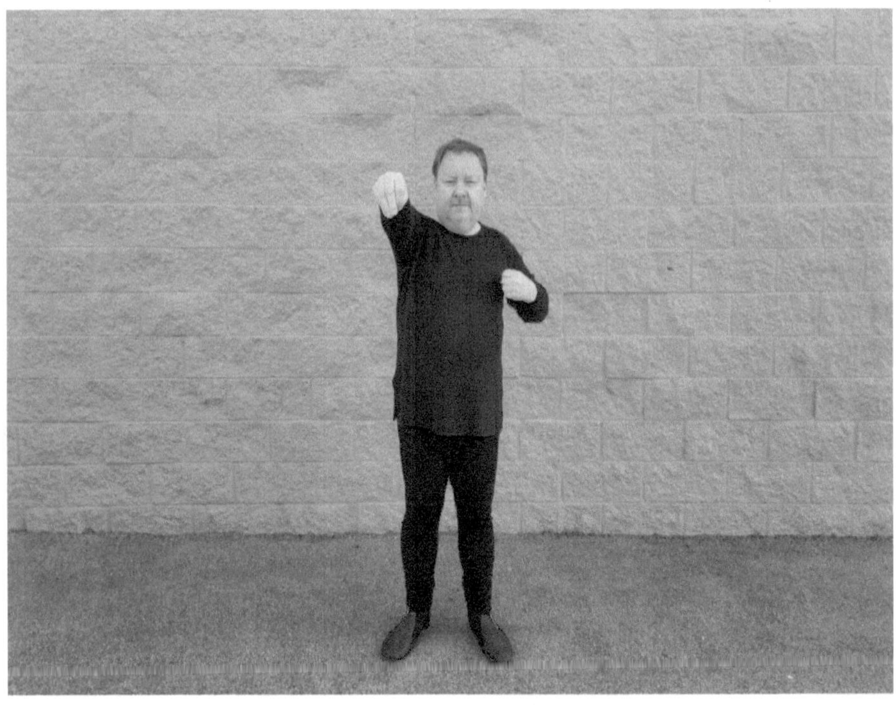

Figure 29 - The Hermit holds a lantern in the right hand and a staff in the left. After you complete this series of poses with your right hand, you will switch and do the series with your left hand leading.

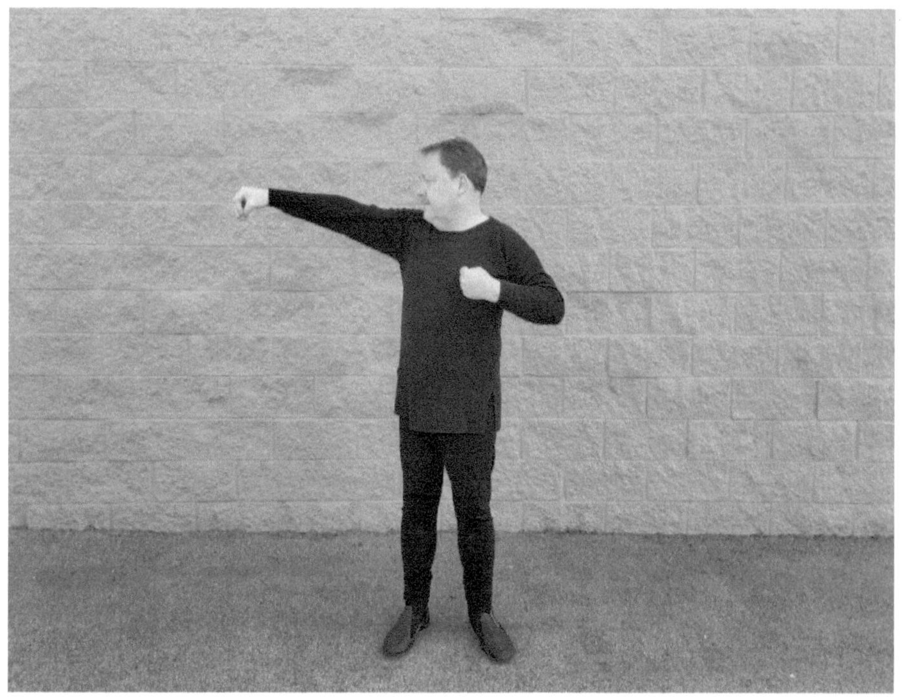

Figure 30 – A quarter turn to the right. You will make all the turns to the right and then will repeat all the movements on the left, too.

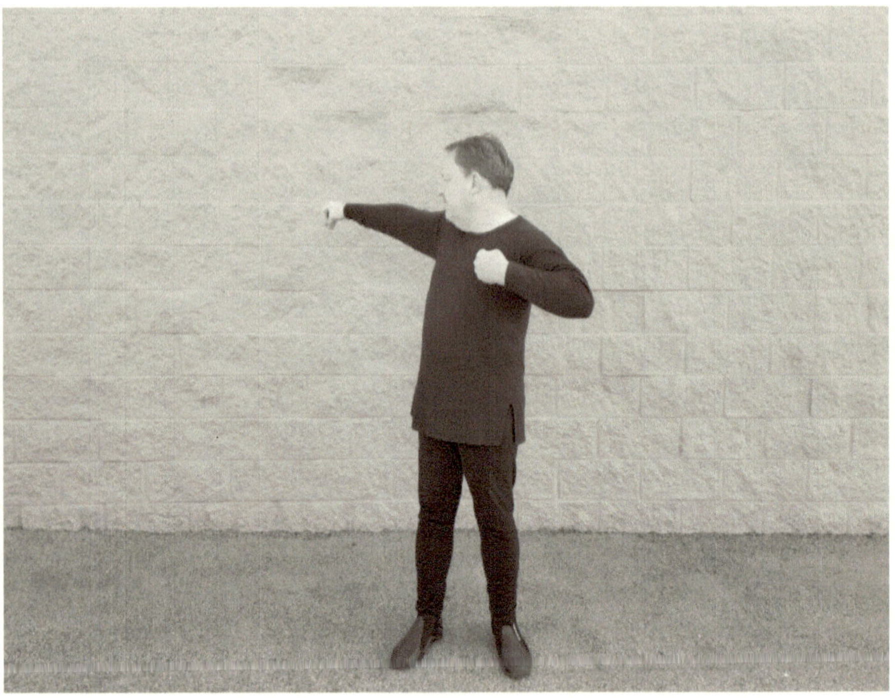

Figure 31 – The Hermit swings the lantern as far back as he can, nearly a full turn to the back, and takes a look.

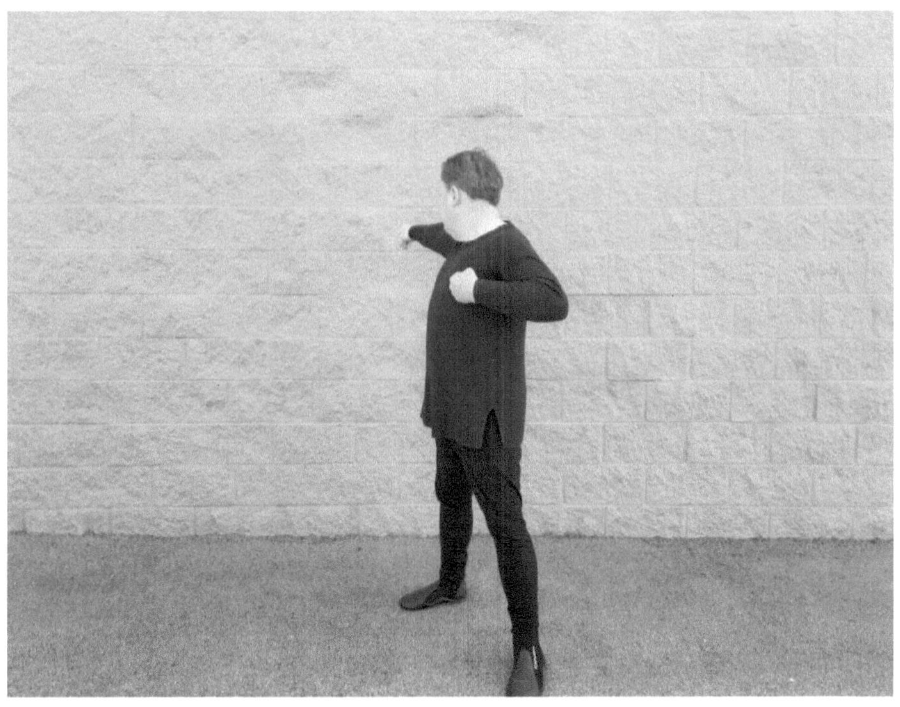

Figure 32 – The Hermit takes a step back and swings his lantern all the way back into the deep, dark recesses of the past. He will bring the light back to the front, bringing the past into the light of today.

△△△

THE WHEEL OF FORTUNE

Chapter 11

You do not know what each day will bring you.
Chances are, nothing momentous will happen.
Then again, you might get hit by lightning
or win the lottery.

THE WHEEL OF FORTUNE is all about destiny, luck, and fate! There are so many depictions and associations with the wheel of fortune. The wheel can have many varieties, different spoke arrangements, different placements, varied creatures, words and symbolism. Sometimes, the wheel is shown as a blindfolded person, blind fortune, that is spinning the wheel. Whatever the imagery, this card is about the circular actions, reactions and (possible) destinies we all experience.

Clasp both hands together straight above your head, and imagine you are holding a huge marker or pen. Beginning at the top, you will "draw" a full circle, with both hands still together, moving to the right, then leaning down, to the left and then back to the top. Imagine a full, round circle. You will make this circle three times.

At the bottom of each circle that you make, there is a little moment in the movement where you can let go of any pressure or tension in your arms. That little moment is a time where your arms hang free and you can feel a weightless freedom from destiny before you finish scribing the wheel. And back to home position.

Movement/Energy Focus:

Arms, Hands, Shoulders, Waist, Torso

GO A LITTLE DEEPER:

This is the halfway point in the 22 Forms of Tarot-Chi™. The Wheel of Fortune has spun for us all, and our journey has taken us from the innocence of beginning as The Fool, through turning away from it all as The Hermit. This is the story of life. But there is more to come. As I am drawing that circle during these poses, I always take the little pause at the bottom of the circle to think about the passing of time. It moves so quickly, the wheel of life spins on and on. Be fully engaged in what life brings to you! Always be learning, always be open to what the wheel brings to you.

Sometimes, life brings great things, and sometimes not so much. Like the Hermit, who turned away from it all, at times, we might curse the wheel and what life brings us. But, I have a perspective that every experience in life is a learning experience – either I am the teacher or I am the student. But it is always about learning. This is what I remember at the bottom of every circle of The Wheel of Fortune.

△△△

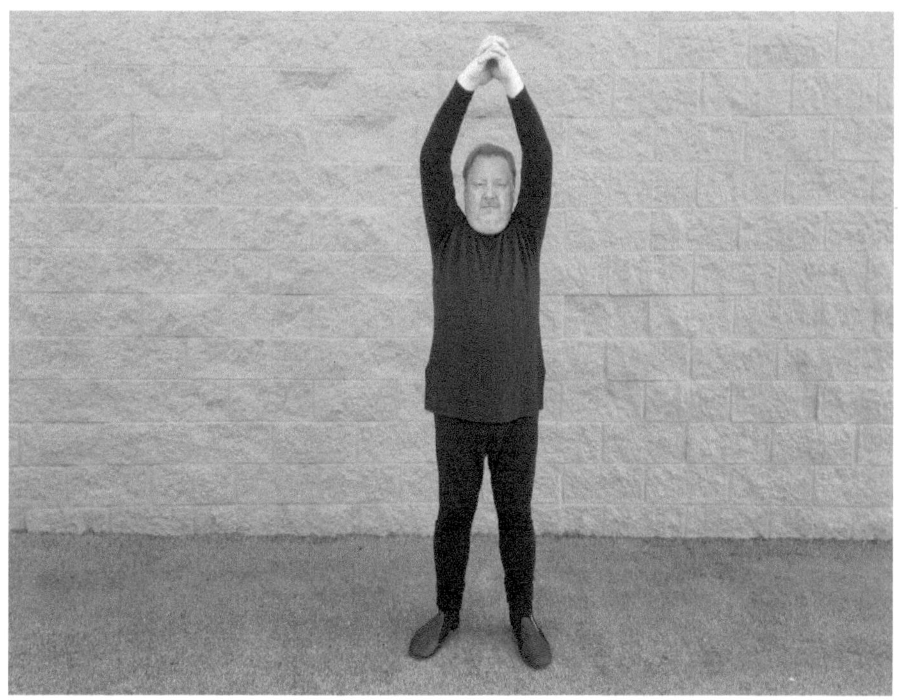

Figure 33 - Arms up in the air, hands clasped together. Imagine you are holding a huge pen or pencil. Keep your hands clasped and make a big circle pattern, beginning from the upper right.

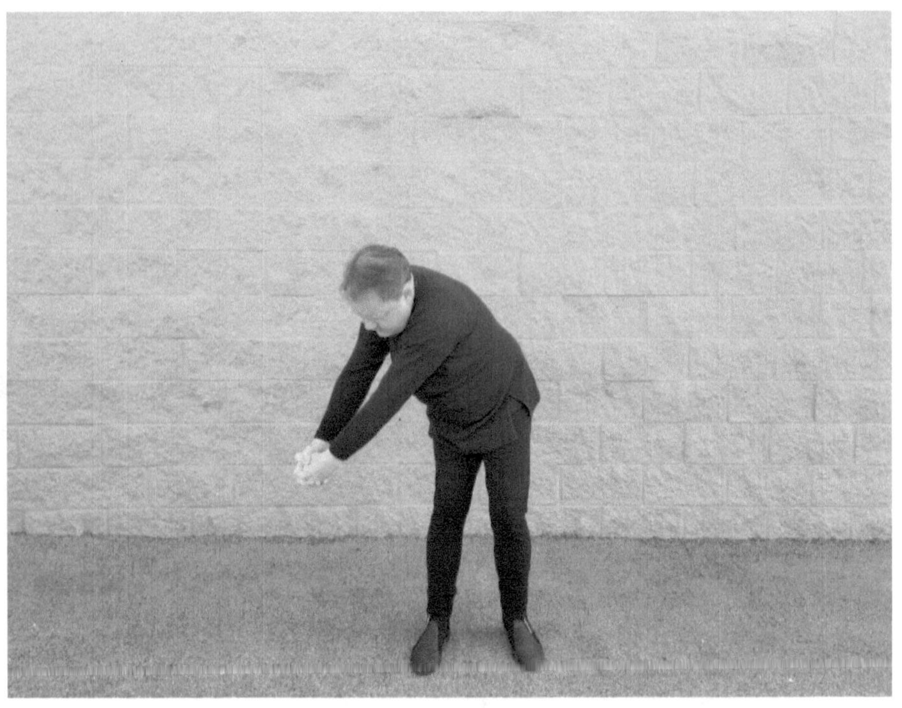

Figure 34 – Nearing the bottom of the circle.

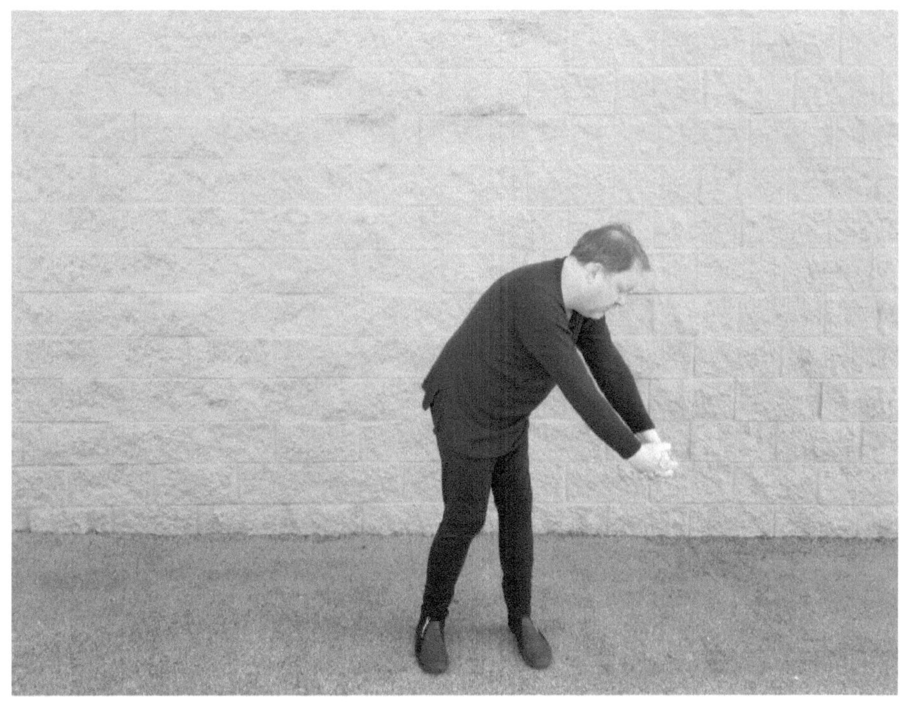

Figure 35- You will make 3 complete circles.

△△△

STRENGTH

Chapter 12

Looking at your problems directly can be frightening. But it can also give you strength, courage, and confidence to face anything.

STRENGTH is all about the will, the choice to face the difficult aspects of life. Often, this card shows a woman holding a lion's jaws shut, although sometimes she is shown riding the creature or just touching it. Think of the symbolism of enlightenment and mental strength over cravings and addictions.

This is my battle card. Do you need to take back control over an issue or two in your life? Me, too! To channel our inner warrior, our inner Boudicca, we will start this series of poses with the arms stretched out in front with palms up.

(Don't know about Boudicca? Go look her up! She was a real person back in the 1st century and led her people to fight back against the oppressive forces of the Roman legions. She sacked Londinium, before it became London. She was fierce!)

Step back with your right foot and swing your right arm down and back, making a large circle. As you swing the right arm back and around to the front, you will bring your right palm to touch the left palm. This symbolizes the closing of the lion's mouth. What is YOUR lion? It can be any issue that you need to take control over.

Stay in that position with your feet, and repeat the hand motion three times. At the third, return your foot to the starting position. Then switch and do this three times with the left hand making the circle and the right palm up.

(Strength and Justice, cards 8 and 11, are sometimes switched in some decks. There are astrological issues here, and Tarot designers make those decision for the deck they are creating. Either card in either position is fine. If your deck switches them, then feel free to switch the position in your exercise routine.)

Movement/Energy Focus:

Hands, Arms, Shoulders, Torso, Hips, Legs

GO A LITTLE DEEPER:

As you practice these movements, remember what you are taking charge over. Remember what you are battling against. Now, some people believe that naming your problems gives them more power. To speak openly about the negatives and to openly "do battle" with your problems is not giving power to the problems. It is taking back your own personal power as a warrior. As you practice the poses for this card, I want you to SEE yourself shutting the mouth of the lion. See the lion as the representative of whatever challenges you have. See yourself as powerful and taking charge. Implant that powerful image in your mind and make it so! (And go read a story about Boudicca or your favorite real superhero.)

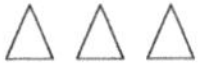

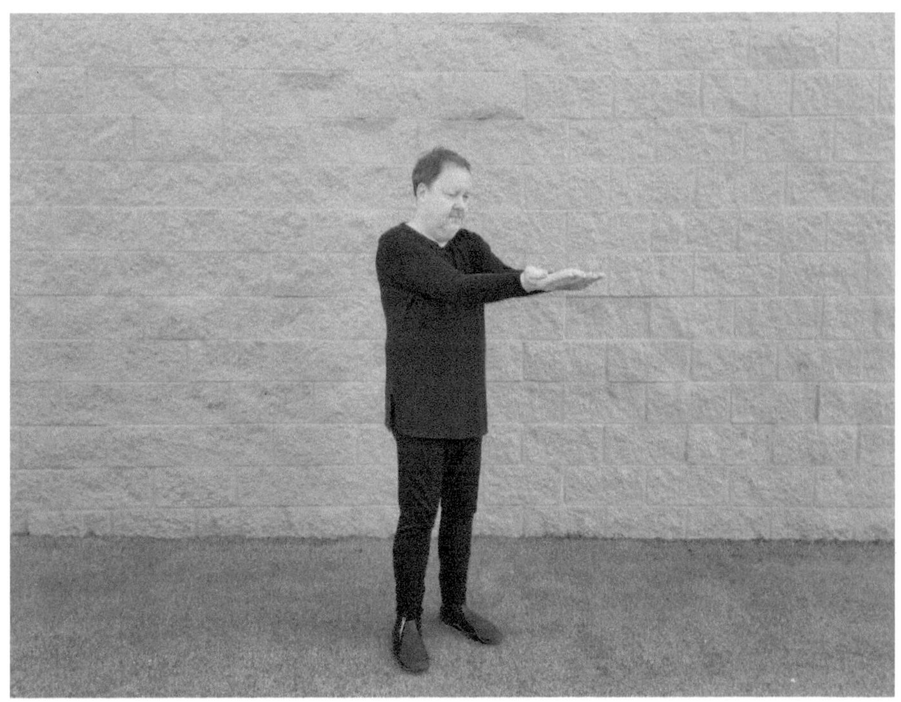

Figure 36 - Arms fully extended in front. From here you will step back with the right foot. Complete the series and then you will step back with your left foot.

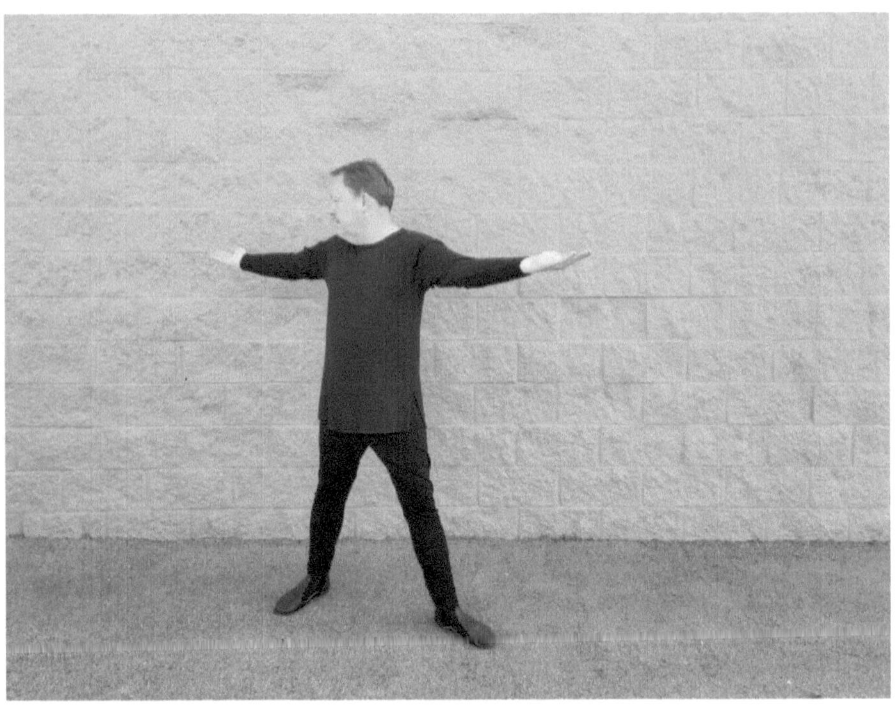

Figure 37 – As you step back with the right foot, your right arm will also go back. Make a large arc and swing the arm forward to shut the mouth of the lion. Repeat 3 times.

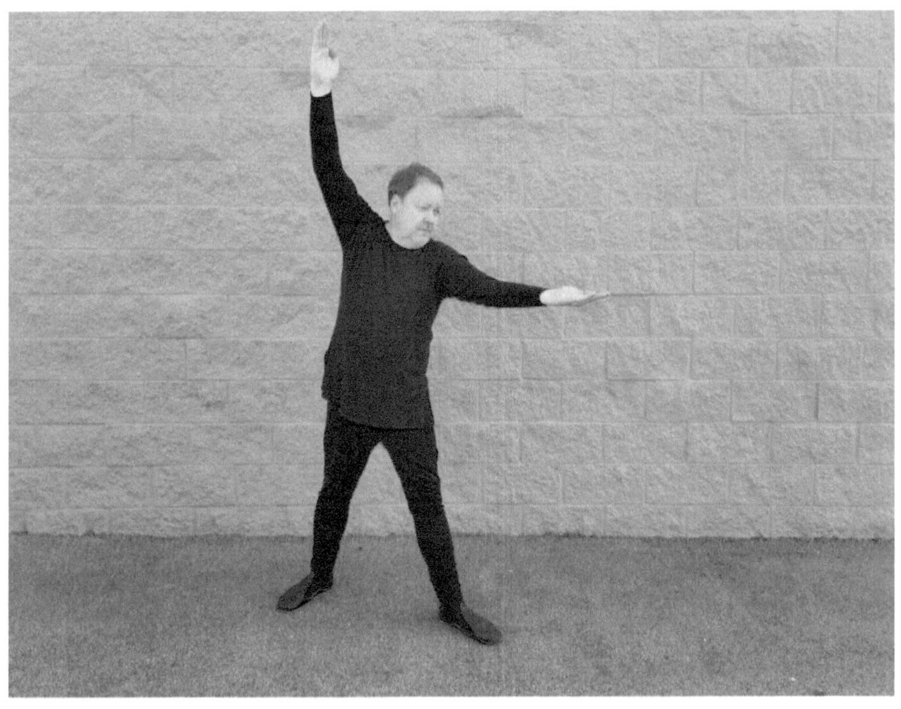

Figure 38 – Continuing the arm movement as you move to shut the mouth of the lion.

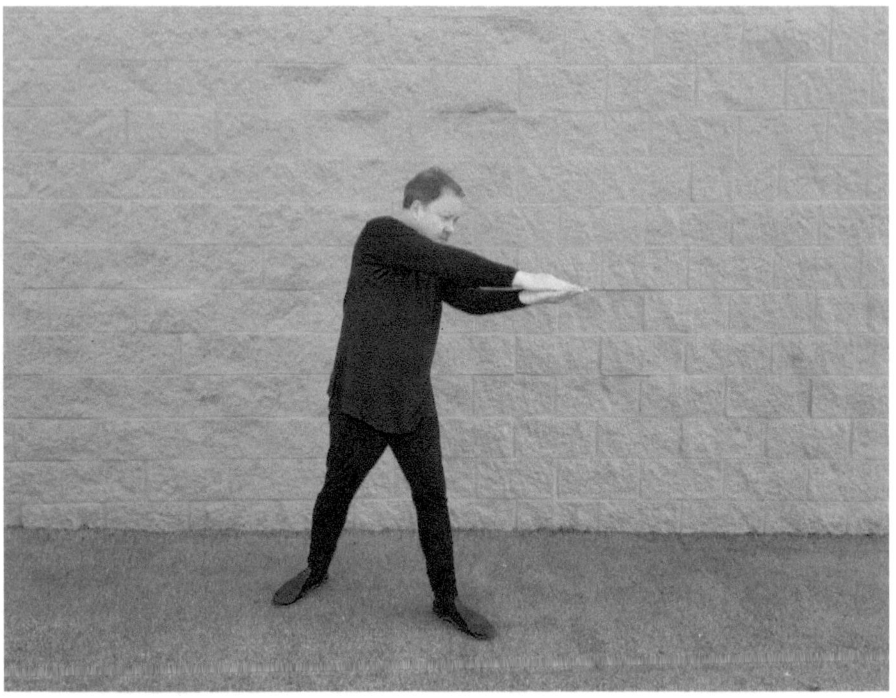

Figure 39 – Shutting the mouth of the lion, showing strength, and taking back control over your own personal issues.

△△△

THE HANGED MAN

Chapter 13

Every action has an equal and opposite reaction - this is a basic law of physics. It is a basic law of human life, too. Every choice you make comes with a sacrifice or repercussion.

THE HANGED MAN often has a serene and peaceful look on his face. He is usually shown hanging upside down by his foot, but it does not look like he is in torment from being punished. It seems as if his upside-down predicament is all about deliberate and chosen self-sacrifice.

This card brings to mind religious concepts throughout the world. There are tales of gods who sacrifice for the good of their followers, think of the Christian Jesus and the Norse god Odin.

To create this series of poses, first raise your arms all the way up and take a deep breath. Exhale fully, and then very slowly bend over at the waist and as far down as possible. If you need to bend your knees, then do so. Or you can just bend all the way over from the waist, keeping your knees straight.

Allow your torso to hang freely. This movement can allow your spine to decompress. It can release pressure in the tissue and fluids between the vertebra. As you are hanging freely, exhale any remaining air. You might hear popping in your back, knees, or even in your ears as you move and flex your joints and muscles.

Inhale slowly as you slowly begin to rise, engaging your core muscles by tightening them and rolling upright one vertebra at a time. Your front thigh muscles will be the first to engage as you rise up. Your stomach and core muscles will be next, and then finally, you will feel the muscles in your back flex as you rise. Your shoulders and then your neck will be the last bit of your body to return to an upright position. Do this full movement twice and then back to home position. (This movement always makes me sigh with relaxation! And it makes my knees pop, too.)

Movement/Energy Focus:

Arms, Shoulders, Waist, Torso, Knees, Spine, Shoulders, Neck

GO A LITTLE DEEPER:

Imagine that you are doing "The Wave" at a ballgame, just do it in super slow motion. When you lift your arms to begin this pose, you can get a deeper stretch by leaning back and really allowing your upper and middle back to stretch. Once you have bent fully over and your upper torso, arms and neck are hanging freely, this will allow your entire spine to decompress. You will then begin rising as slowly as possible.

There is something so incredibly relaxing about this pose for me, that I always take a moment to inhale deeply and sigh after I rise both times. That state of relaxation can be intense, and I enjoy those little moments of blissful relaxation. See if it affects you the same way. This is a time in Tarot-Chi where the action stops completely. Most of the poses are very fluid and the movements just flow from one into the next. But here, we have a full stop, actually, 2 of them. Take the time to breathe deeply and just enjoy the relaxation.

Where this is the slowest section of Tarot-chi, the next series of poses for the next card will be the quickest.

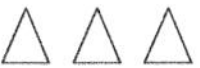

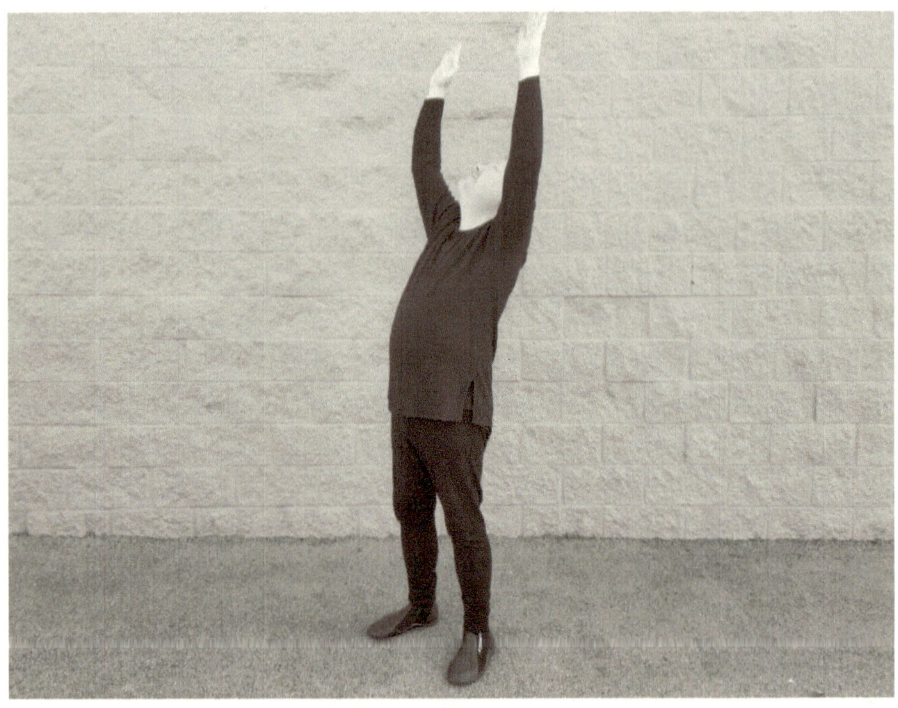

Figure 40 - As you stretch up, take a deep breath and prepare to slowly bend over at the waist, breathing out fully as you do.

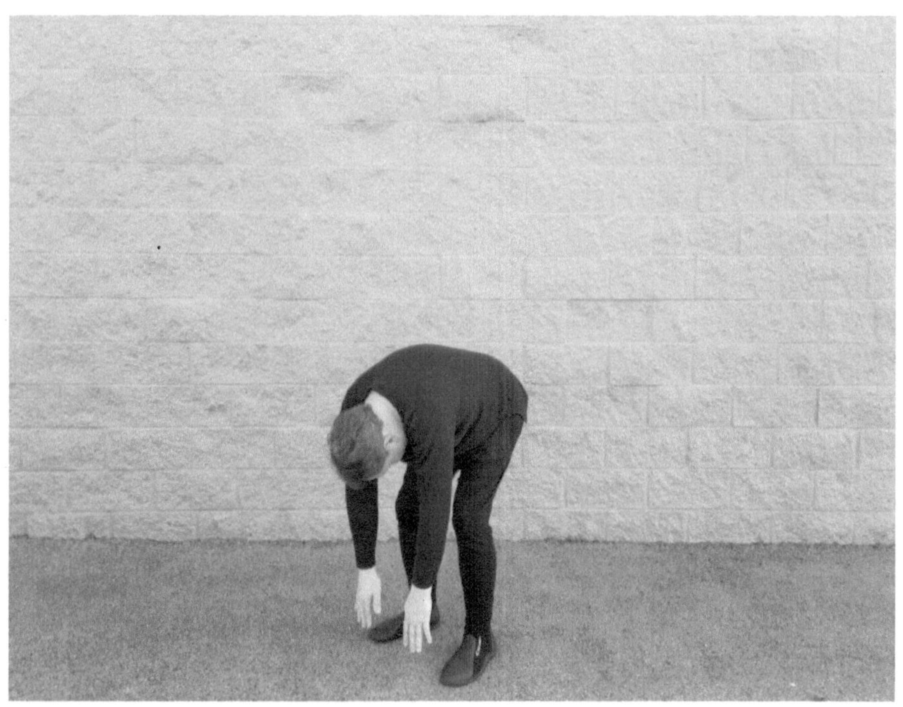

Figure 41- Allow your head, neck and arms to hang freely for several seconds. You are the hanged man.

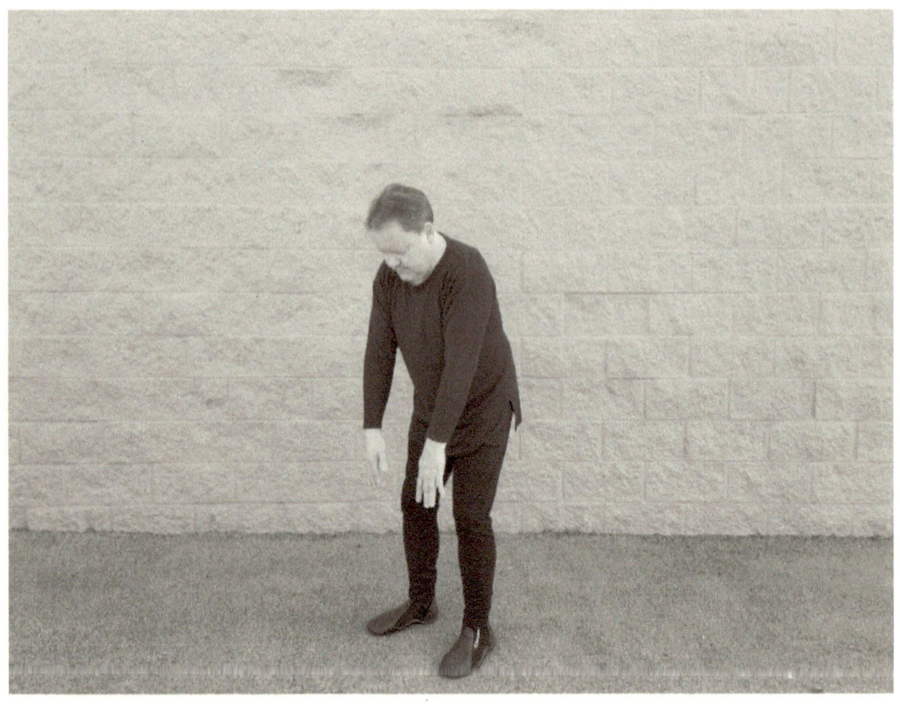

Figure 42 - Slowly roll up, one vertebra at a time, shoulders, neck and head will be last. Remember to breathe in gently.

△△△

DEATH

Chapter 14

Many see death as an end.
But it is not an end, it is a transformation.
The body becomes terra dust;
the soul becomes star dust.

DEATH – so many people are afraid of this card with the Grim Reaper and symbology of decay. I think it is because so many people are truly afraid of death. I once struggled with this fear, too. But so much has happened in my life that I now truly believe in the existence of life after death. I do not know exactly what it will be like, but I will someday.

This card signifies the end and the beginning, a change of what is. This card is about transformation. There can be many different types of transformations in our life. Think of all the wonderful ceremonies that we have that celebrate the changing aspects of life, from graduations to marriages to birth announcements. And yes, death. That is the best way to view death – as a transformation.

Our series of movements will begin with crossing of the arms like scissors cutting a thread, directly in front of you. It is the cutting of the thread of life, the movement of the scythe. That movement is the quickest in the whole series of Tarot-Chi ™. Then you step out with the left foot, heel to toe, in a forty-five-degree angle, while you make the cutting movement with the arms. Come back to the front and do the cutting motion again. Then do that same stepping and cutting movement to the right and back again to the front to finish up with another cutting motion.

The movement changes now as the right foot steps back, and as you turn to the right side, you pull back with your right arm and then extend it fully to the side. Your left foot will still be facing forward, while your right foot is at a 90-degree angle to it. You will be standing in a modified Vitruvian Man pose. You look to the right and then look up. In a single motion, while you bring your right arm in an arc to the front you also bring your right foot back to the beginning position. The right hand goes palm up, signifying transformation.

And now do the same series of poses on the left side. The left hand will go up at the end, signifying transformation. Back to home position. (This is a complex series of movements for this pose, so please discuss this with your instructor or follow along on YouTube and/or the video.)

Movement/Energy Focus:

Arms, Hands, Shoulder, Torso, Legs, Feet

GO A LITTLE DEEPER:

At the beginning of this pose, during the crossed arm movements signifying the cutting of the cord of life, the movements are very quick and sharp. I truly always imagine a "snicker-snack" sound. This comes directly from a line in the poem "Jabberwocky" by Lewis Carroll. Go read it and see what you think.

When you are stepping back with one arm fully extended behind you, make sure you also turn your head. Keep your vision on the arc of the arm as it comes back to the front. This will give you an opportunity for a great neck stretch.

Why are we afraid of death? Are YOU afraid of death? Most people are, and it has been presented in religious groups and movies as a terrifying thing. But what are we really afraid of? Non-existence? Or punishment? IF you believe in the existence of the soul, or spirit, or something that exists beyond the physical body, then death is just another part of your existence, it is just a transformation. It is just another great experience for each of us! And if you believe that the Divine nature is one of love, then there is no punishment that you need to be afraid of.

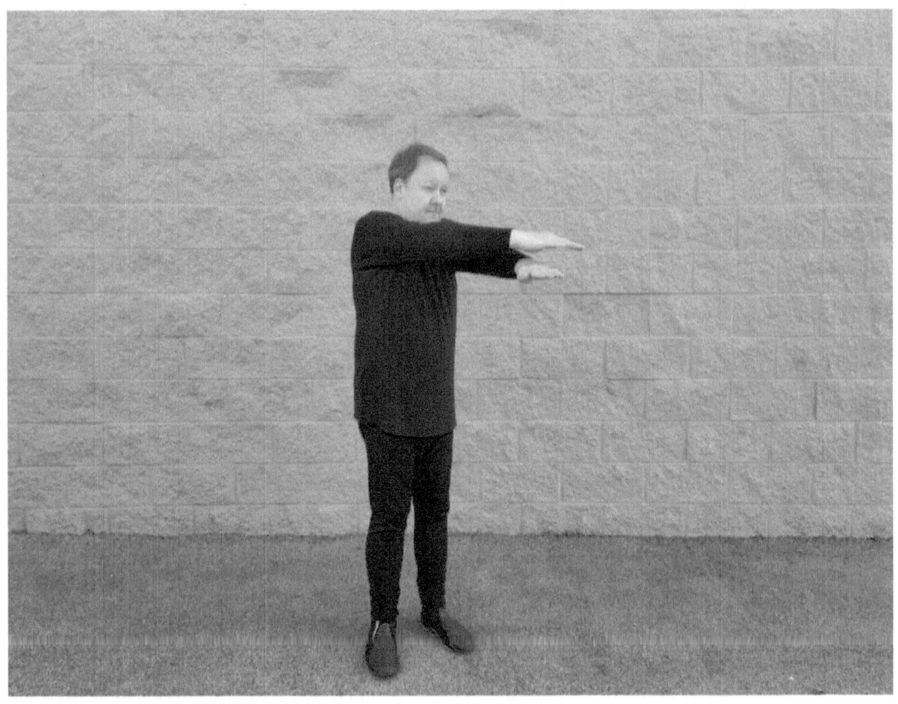

Figure 43 – Your arms will cross in front of you, like scissors or crossed scythes. You will make this crossing motion 5 times.

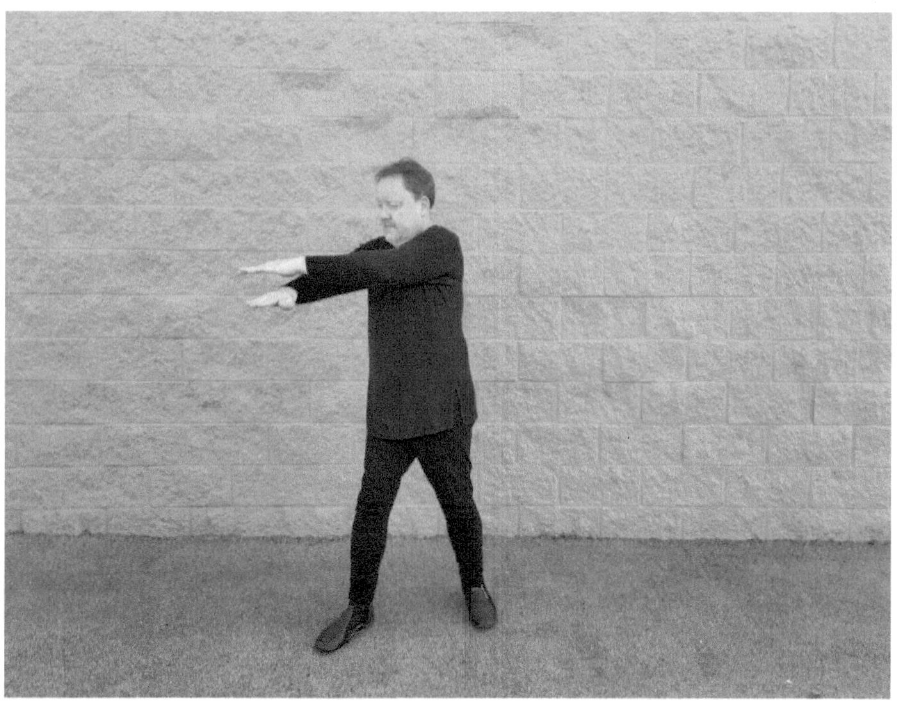

Figure 44 - The cutting motions are made to both the right and left sides, alternating with motions directly in front.

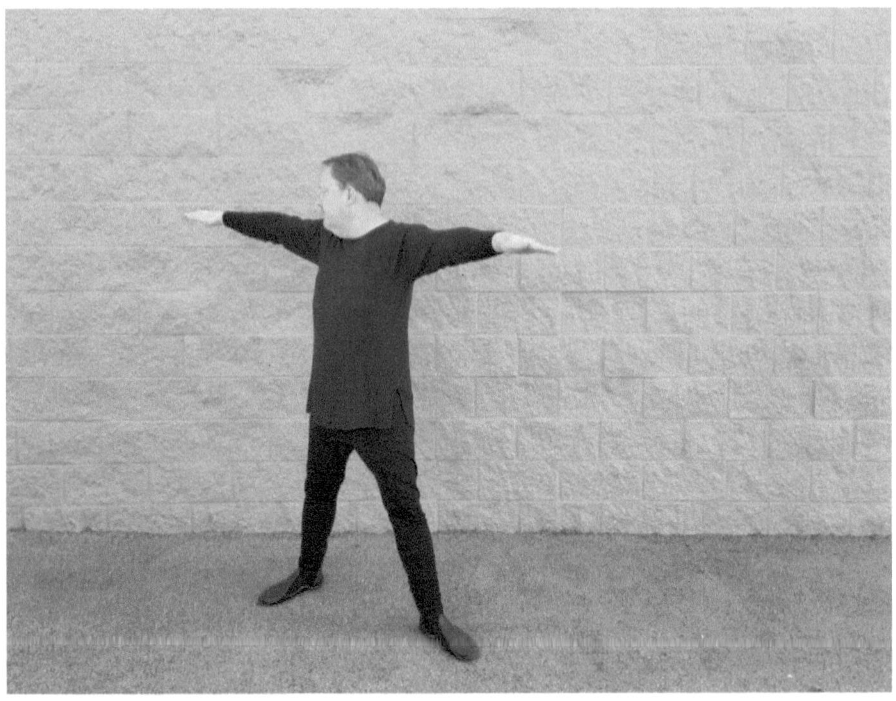

Figure 45- Right arm extends back as right leg steps back. You will complete this series of poses, and then repeat with the other leg and arm.

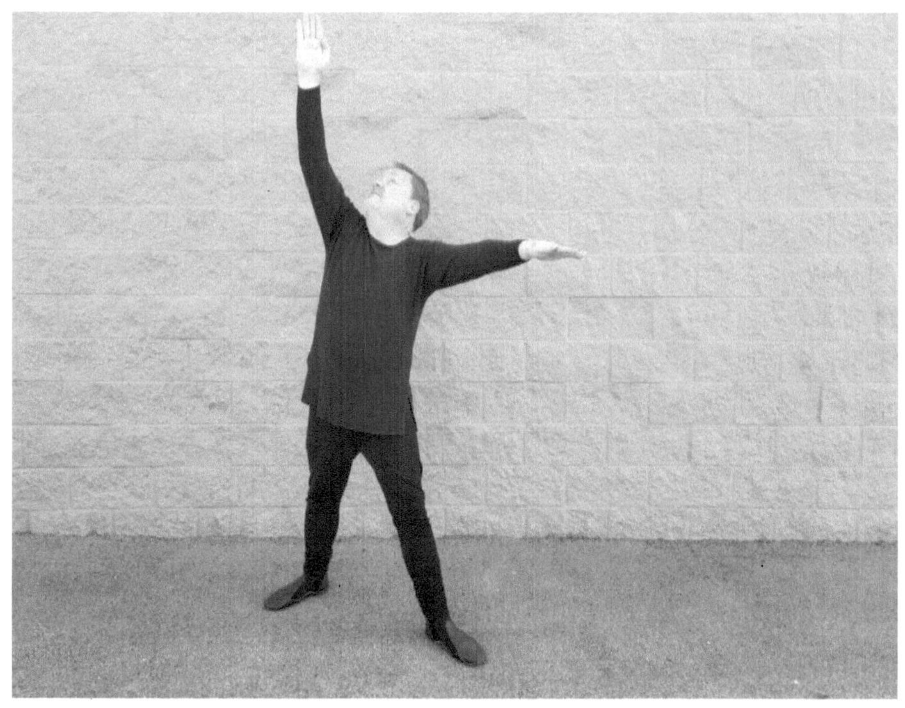

Figure 46 – The arc of life, with the arm coming up and over. You look up and over, too.

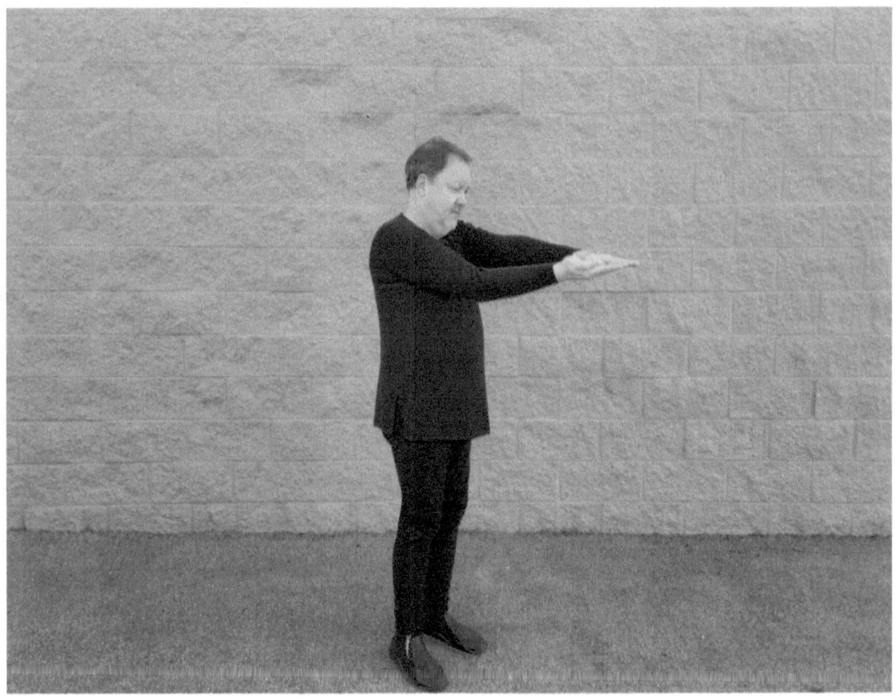

Figure 47 - Pose ends by bringing the foot back to the front along with the hands. One hand will be palm up, signifying death as transition. You will repeat the motions with the other foot and hand.

△△△

TEMPERANCE

Chapter 15

Life is a balancing act; enjoy the
finest things in life, but don't overindulge.
Mixing water with wine was seen as a way to
drink alcohol, but not to excess.
Perhaps this is why we do not eat dessert first?

TEMPERANCE is also known as frugality or moderation. This card is typically shown as a woman or an angel. She is often shown pouring liquid from one cup into another, or possibly pouring liquid out of the cups. Often, the figure holding the two cups is standing with one foot on water and the other foot on the land.

We will begin by shifting all of our weight onto the right leg. When you do this, the left hip naturally lowers. Then lifting the left leg and knee high, we will place the left leg back on the ground. We will then shift all of our weight onto the left leg. The right hip will naturally lower. Then lift the right leg and knee high, placing them back on the ground. Now, our feet are symbolically on the land and in the water.

Your arms go out to the sides, again taking the Vitruvian Man position. With the arms still extended, slowly bring them towards each other in front of you. While you do this, you might feel a tremendous compression and concentration of energy. This whole exercise system has been created so that you can experience and sense the energy that flows in and around your body. So, try to focus on feeling the energy compress as your arms come together.

Imagine you are holding two cups in your hands. You will start symbolically pouring liquid back and forth from one cup to the other. Make each pour in a larger and larger arc, until your arms are fully extended with each pour. Use this time to move and twist your wrists. Then bring the arms back in, reducing the arc, until your hands are back in the beginning position.

It usually takes about 18 twists of the hands and wrists to get out and back into the home position. You can make it as few as 16 or as many as 20.

<u>Movement/Energy Focus:</u>

Hips, Knees, Legs, Shoulders, Arms, Wrists, Hands

<u>GO A LITTLE DEEPER:</u>

The movement of shifting the imaginary liquid back and forth in the cups needs to stay focused in the upper half of your body. Don't swing the cups so widely that you are making arcs all the way down to your knees. The main movement focus is on the shoulders and wrists.

Since your feet do not move much during this series of poses, you can choose to squat and create movement/tension in your thighs and core while you are swinging the wrists and arms. Because you have stepped out and expanded your stance, this can be a challenging position to maintain. You can add a squat to any of the poses that are upper torso focused.

The energy of this series of poses might remind you of The Empress, where you gathered up a ball of Earth energy. But the true association here is with the Lovers. You are combining forces in the two cups. As you transfer the imaginary liquid between the cups (I always think of them like goblets – holy grails) think of what loving forces you are combining in your life. Think of what you WANT to combine. Maybe it is increased income with a better job. Maybe it is a loving partner and some fabu bedroom fun that you want to combine. Whatever it is, imagine how you are bringing the good things in life to you and how you are combining them into one great experience.

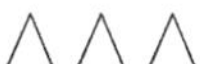

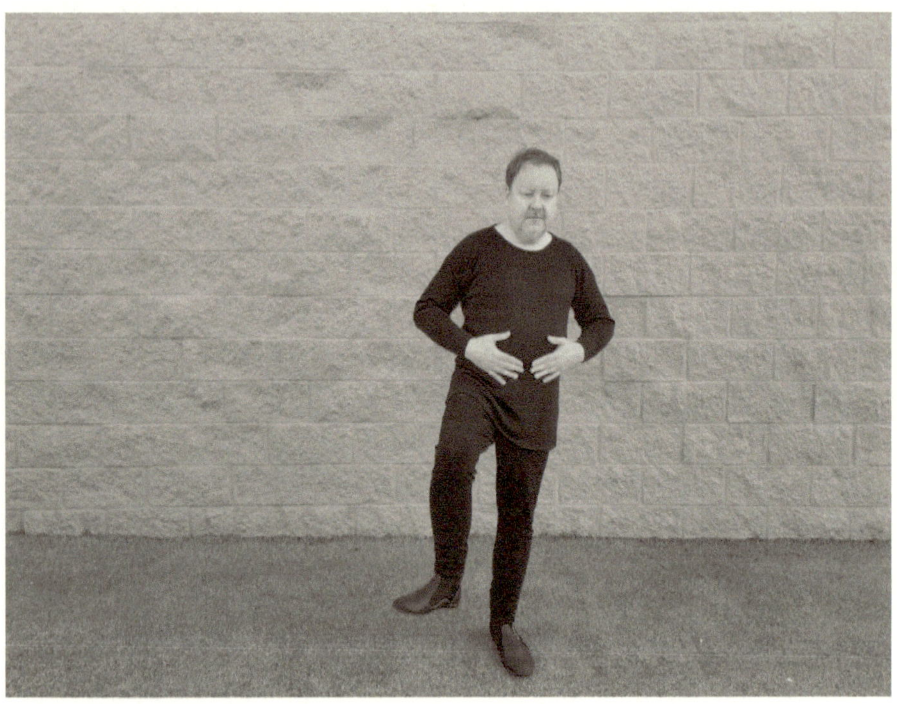

Figure 48 - As you shift your full weight onto one leg, you lift the other as high as possible before placing it back on the ground. Then shift all your weight to the other hip. And repeat the movement.

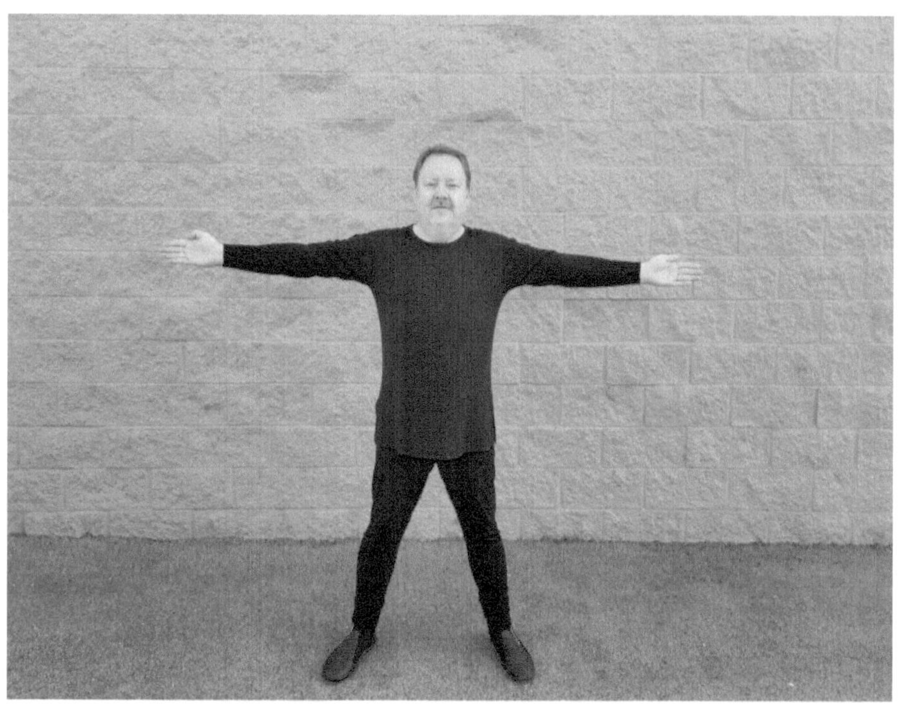

Figure 49 - Standing in the Vitruvian Man position.

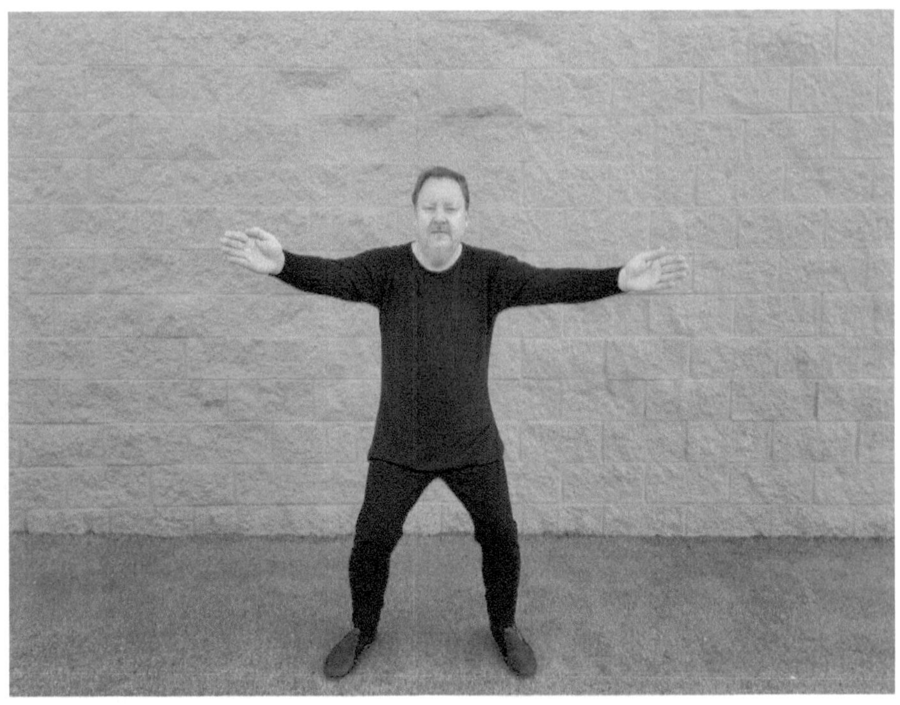

Figure 50 – Squat and bring your arms in toward the center of your body.

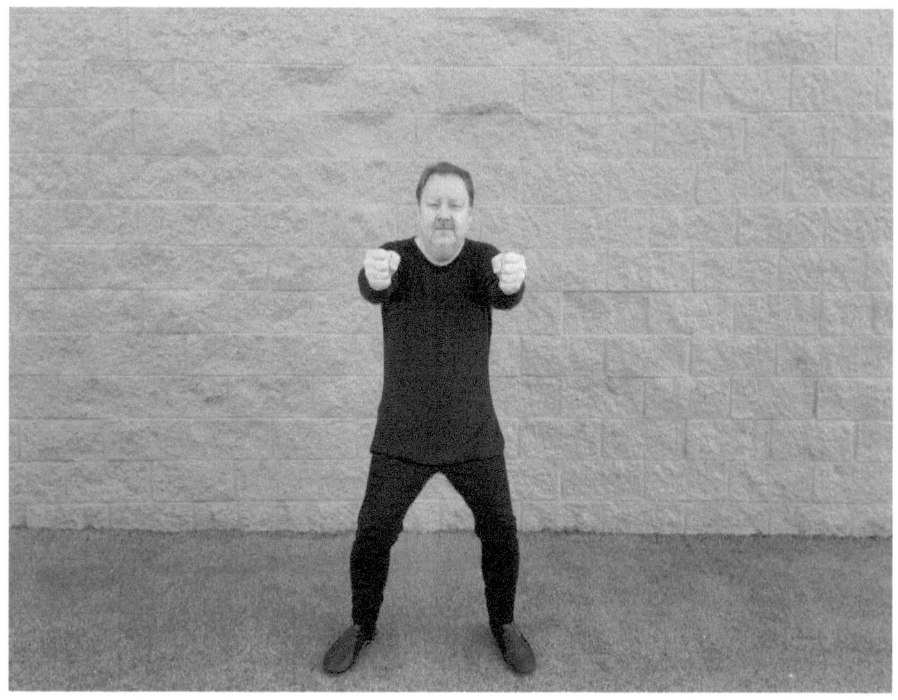

Figure 51 – As your arms come to the front and center, imagine you are holding two cups. We will be pouring back and forth and combining the ingredients. What are you combining in your life? What do you WANT to be combining?

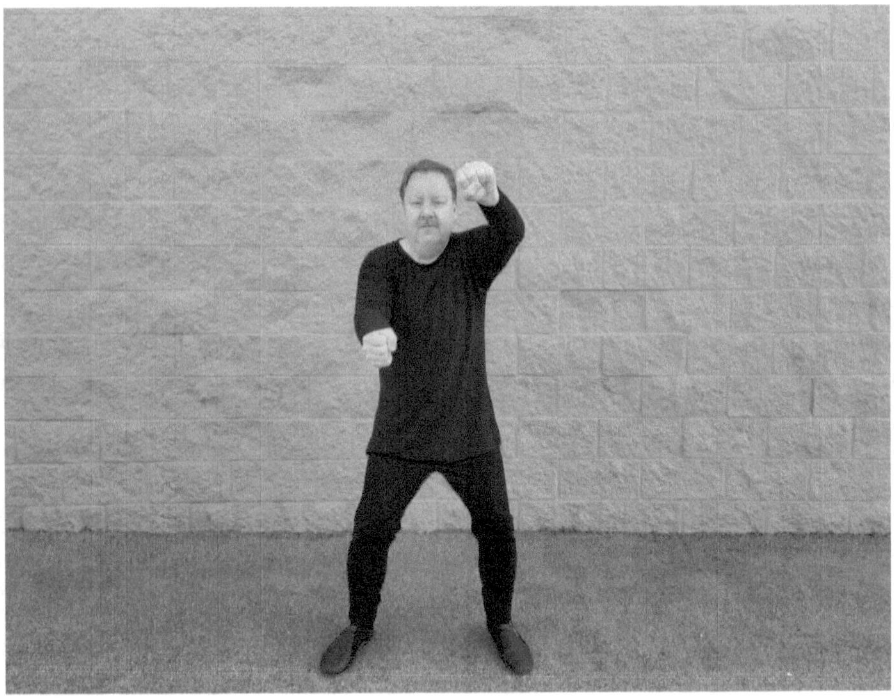

Figure 52 - Pouring back and forth from one glass to the other. Twist your wrists and hands in a widening arc.

△△△

THE DEVIL

Chapter 16

Growing up, I was taught to believe that the devil was real and so was hell. Now, I believe that people can experience hell right here on Earth. The true enemy is not some hobgoblin with horns, but our own thoughts, negative emotions, and addictions.

THE DEVIL is often shown as a combination of human and animal parts – a man's face with goat horns, bat wings, raptor feet and usually a pentagram scribed somewhere on his body. He is hideous; definitely the substance of nightmares. The card often shows a naked couple chained to the Devil's throne or pedestal. This can be a representation of seduction, lust and obsession, or possibly even fear, addiction or bondage.

We are going to release the chains that are holding the couple. As we release their chains, we will also focus on releasing our own! This is my favorite series of poses in the whole Tarot-Chi ™ system. It is about acknowledging your chains, releasing them, and finding freedom. This is powerful imagery to change your life!

Bring your hands up beside your head. This might look like horns, but it represents shielding your thoughts and mind from negative influences. Then, you will step to the left, as you move your arms to the left. You will reach out as if to grasp a chain. You will yank on the chain twice and then let go. As you step back to the center position, you bring your hands back up again to your head. You will then switch to the right side and make the same motions.

Finally, you are going to repeat the two motions again, but with one large difference. When you yank the chains on each side, you will then let go of the chains, open your arms and hands wide to release the prisoners! Do this on the left, and then hands back to the center and up to your head. Do this on the right, and then hands back to the center and up to your head again. This last time, your hands will not go back to the home position, but you will transition directly into the next form.

Movement/Energy Focus:

Hands, Arms, Hips, Torso, Legs, Feet

GO A LITTLE DEEPER:

As you step to the right or left and "yank" on the chains in this move, you can make the movement longer and deeper. This will allow you to extend those leg muscles for a greater stretch. If you do extend the step out, you may need to take 2 steps to get back into the central position. Just adjust as needed.

As you begin the second round of steps to the side, when you open your hands to release the chains holding the captives or minions, this move is a meditation on our own personal demons, our own chains that need to be released. There is an old folk saying, "Mend your own heart before you try to mend others." It is a good thing to want to help others, but do not judge others and their predicaments. Mend yourself first. During this move, focus on what you need to release, what is holding you back, and how you can heal moving forward.

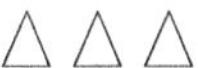

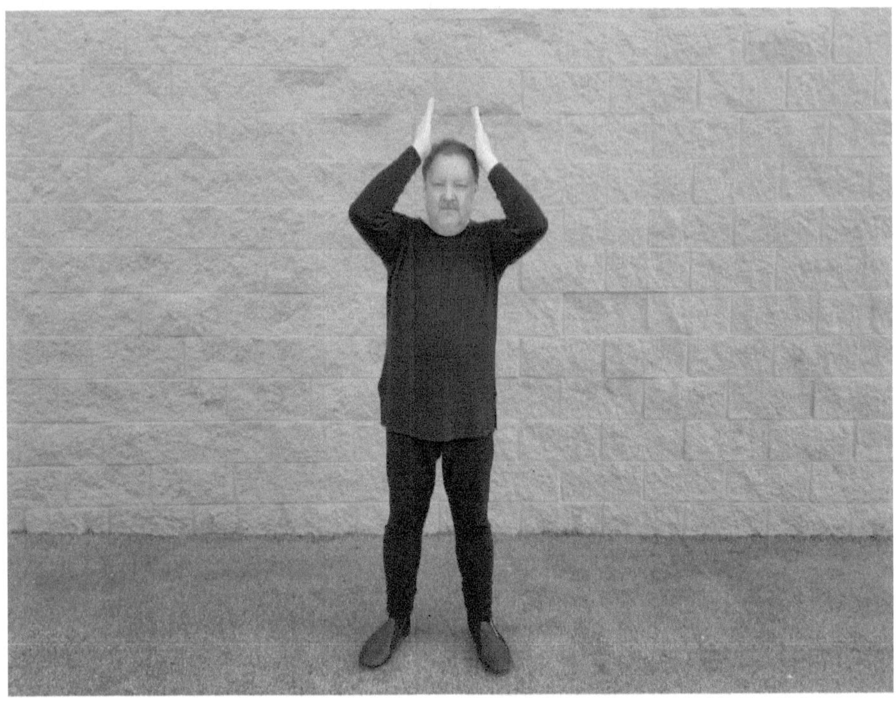

Figure 53 - It might look like the classic horns of a devil, but it symbolizes the decision to protect your mind, body and spirit from negative forces.

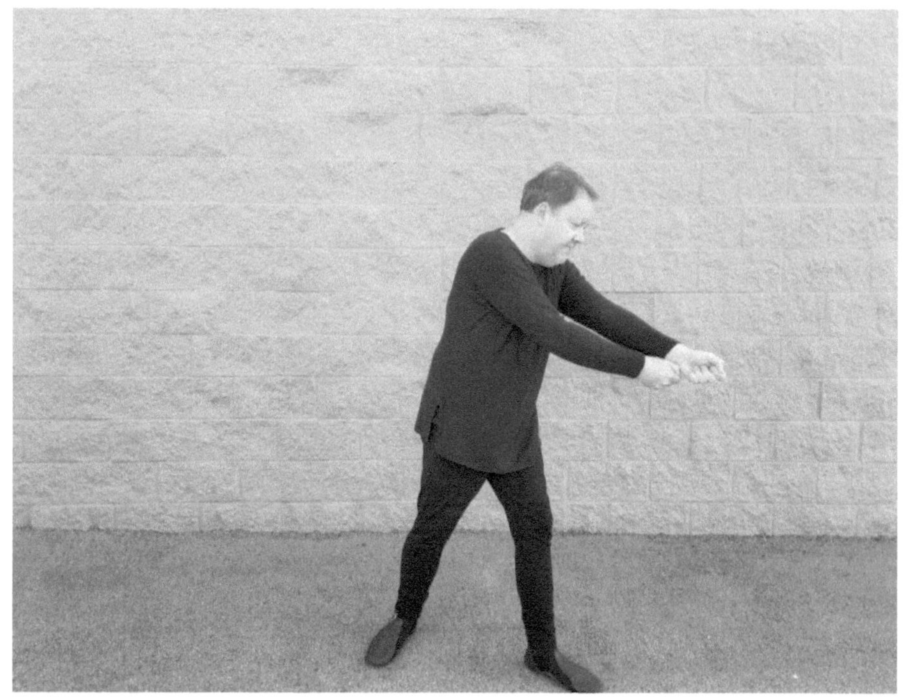

Figure 54 - We tug on the chains that are binding the captives.

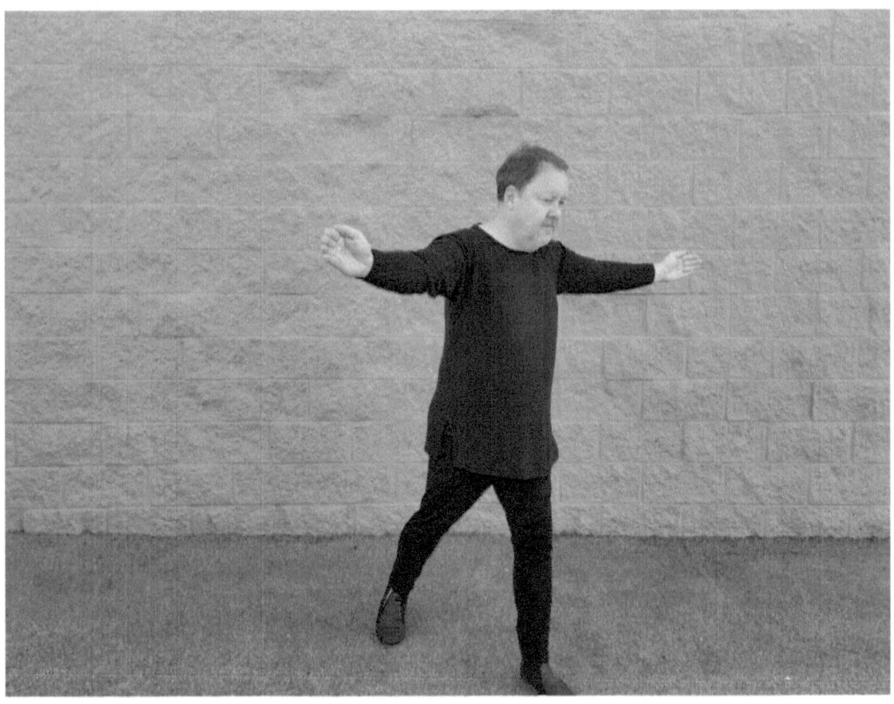

Figure 55 - My favorite move in all of Tarot-Chi ™ - this is where we release the captives. What is binding you in life? What can you release from your life?

△△△

THE TOWER

Chapter 17

Are you afraid of heights?
The higher the tower, the greater the fall.
But the higher the tower, the greater the view.

THE TOWER is suddenly struck by lightning. It burns down as everyone falls. It is a frightening concept, and this card shows the possibility of sudden and destructive change. The Tower can be seen as a card of danger. There is a crisis and calamity! But burning down the tower can also lead to a new and better structure being built. So, the card can also be about liberation from the old ways of thinking and doing.

From the last section of the last pose, your hands were beside your head. Now, raise your arms directly above your head to symbolize a tower. Angle your arms to the left and bring them quickly up and down twice to signify a lightning strike. Do the same on the right side. Return your arms to the center, extended above your head.

Take one full step back with your left foot first, and then your right foot. Then bend over from the waist and let your hands touch your toes. Bend your knees if needed, or keep them straight if you can. This shows how the tower has fallen.

Stand back up and repeat the entire sequence again. Only on the second time, instead of rising as the tower, you will rise with arms outstretched in front. You will take one big step forward, leading with your right foot. Squat down slightly and place your outstretched arms in front of you to catch those who are falling. And back to home position.

Movement/Energy Focus:

Arms, Shoulders, Waist, Torso, Hips, Thighs, Knees

GO A LITTLE DEEPER:

You have the opportunity to make a long step backwards and forwards with this set of poses. When you bend over, make it slow and steady. Any bending from the spine should be done gently so as to stretch but not damage. You can also squat deeply at the end and that will extend the stretch of this pose.

The card is about sudden change, which can be devastating. Ask anyone living in Oklahoma who has suffered through a tornado - one minute you have a house, and the next minute you don't. Natural disasters test human nature in some interesting ways. You will find heroic rescues where neighbors help each other, or our military forces save lives. Then again, you will find looters who go in and try to take advantage of someone else's pain. At some point in your life, you will have the opportunity to receive help and to offer it. Be kind always, and be appreciative.

When massive change happens, there is an opportunity for massive growth, too. I have always liked to say that, "There is no breakthrough without a breakdown." Good can come from even the worst in life, but sometimes, you just have to make it so.

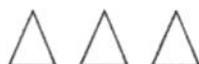

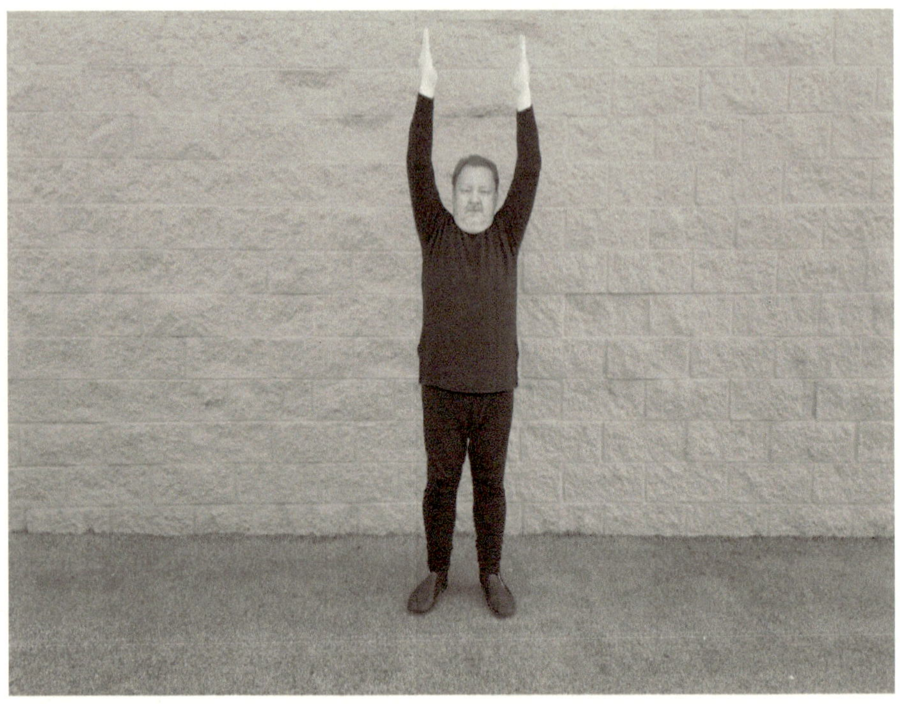

Figure 56 - Straight from the last card, we move directly into the symbology of the Tower.

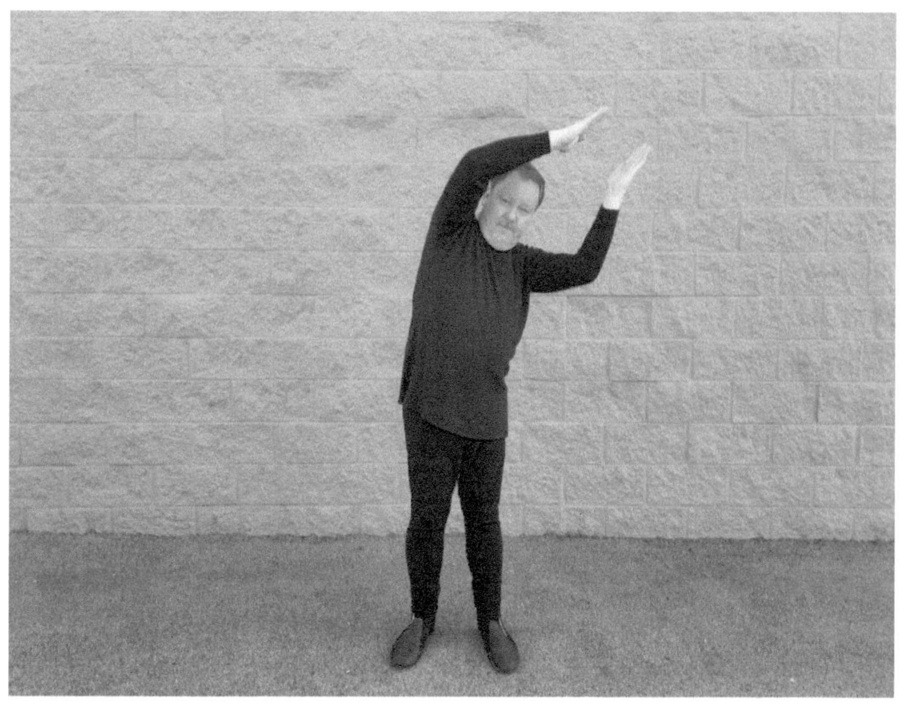

Figure 57 -Lightning strikes from the right.

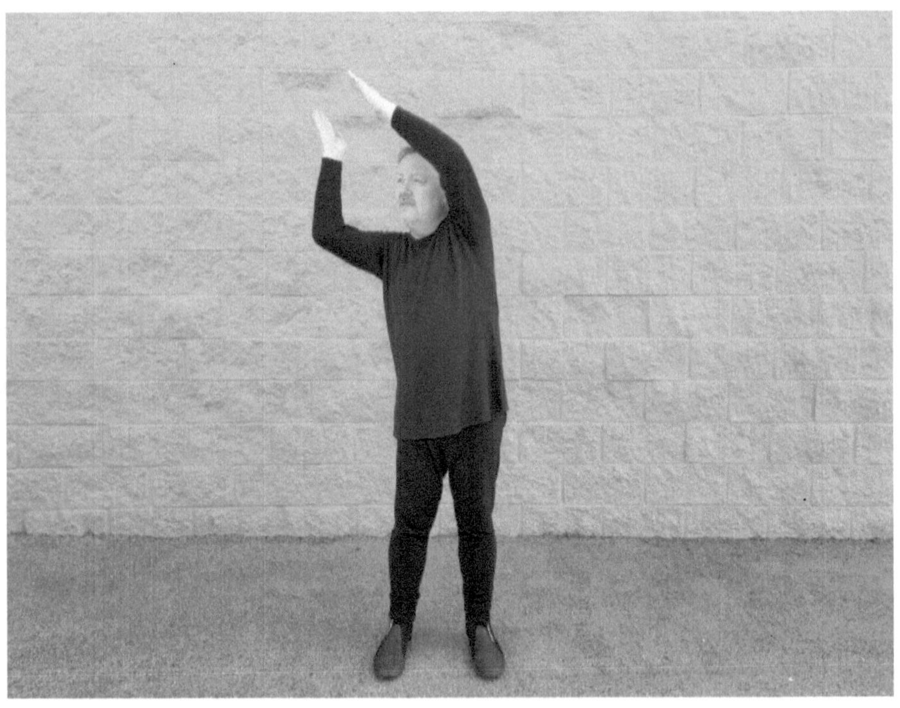

Figure 58 - Lightning strikes from the left

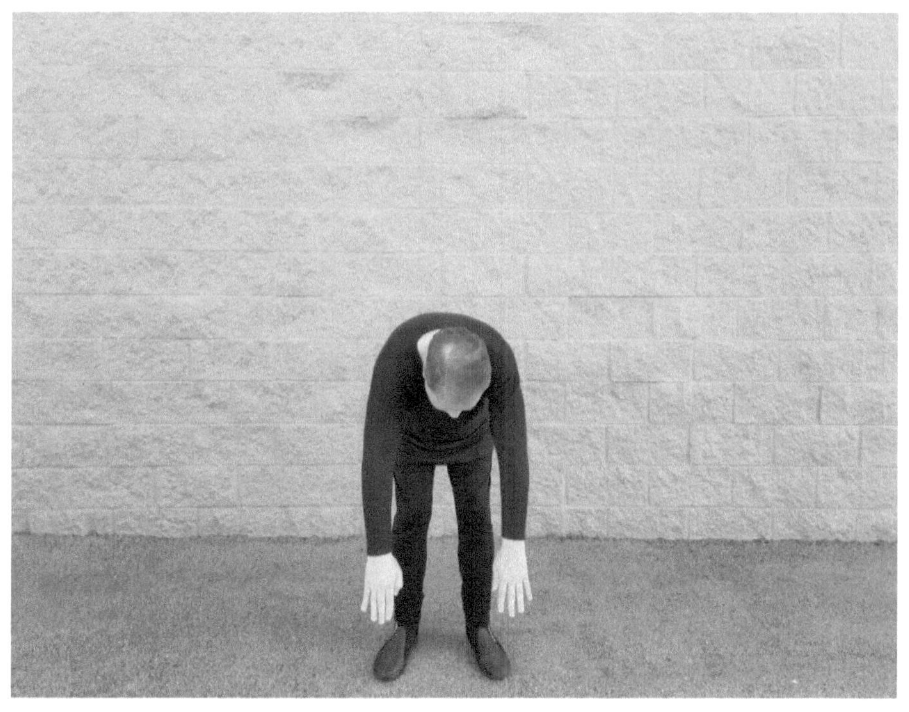

Figure 59 - And we all fall down!

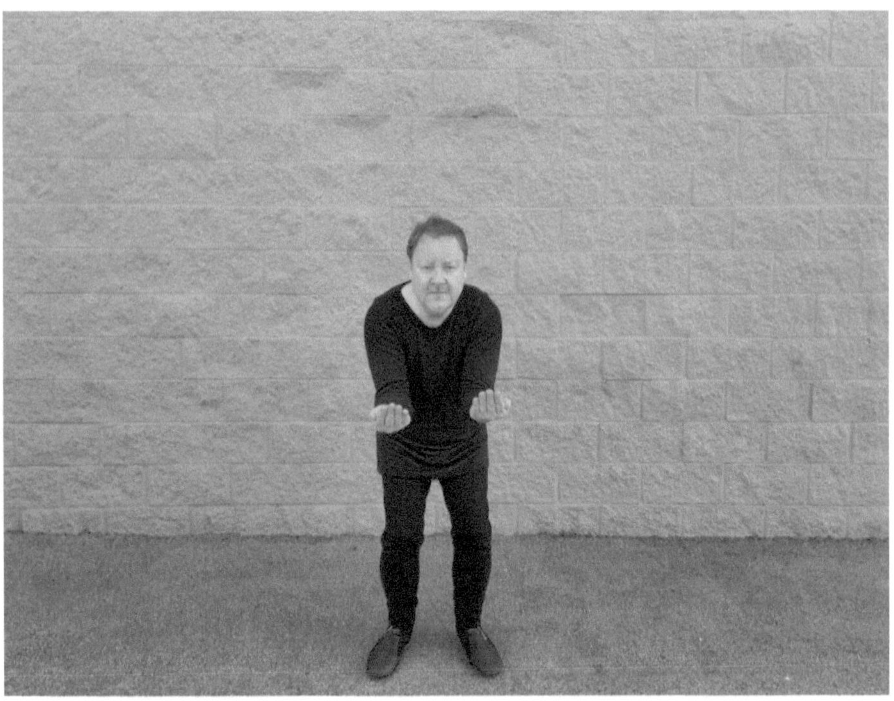

Figure 60 - On the second repetition of this series, instead of standing straight up, lean in to catch those who are falling.

△ △ △

THE STAR

Chapter 18

Only in the deepest dark night of the soul will you be able to see the glorious light of the stars.

THE STAR shines down on a beautiful woman, often naked, as she is kneeling by the water. One foot is in the water and one is on the land. There is a large star above her, showing that she is a divine spirit, and there are usually several smaller stars around. She holds containers of liquid, and is usually shown pouring her blessings from above out on the water and the land. This is one of my favorite images in all Tarot. It is the essence of Divine love and inspiration. The beautiful creature is showering all with the blessings from above. It rains on the just and the unjust.

We will start with the same leg work as in the Temperance card. We will begin by shifting all of our weight onto the right leg. Then lifting the left leg and knee high, we will place the foot back on the floor. We will then shift all of our weight onto the left leg, and lift the right leg and knee high, placing them back onto the floor. Now, our feet are symbolically on the land and in the water.

Reach up to the sky, and as you do, grab two jars of blessings from above. Squat down with the jars in your hand, and begin pouring them out. They are heavy with goodness from above, so you are fully bent over. As the containers empty, they become lighter and you rise while your arms lift back to your sides. Repeat the movement again. Return to home position.

Movement/Energy Focus:

Hips, Legs, Knees, Shoulders, Arms, Hands, Waist, Torso

GO A LITTLE DEEPER:

The "jars of blessings" from above are heavy! Since they are, when you begin pouring them out, they will get lighter. This is a great opportunity to get a full stretch in the outer arm. You are bent over in this pose with your outer arms rotated up towards the sky. Maintain that arm position as you rise, and you will get a great flex in that outer arm.

As you reach up to heaven to receive the jars of blessings, imagine what kind of goodness you are getting. Perhaps one of the jars is full of good things for the people you love, and one of them is filled with the good things in life just for you. What are you receiving from above? And what are you pouring out on others? Use this time to refocus and be thankful for all the little things that you have in your life and all the little extra joys that life brings your way. This is the Tarot-Chi™ equivalent of stopping to smell the roses! Be ye thankful.

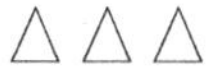

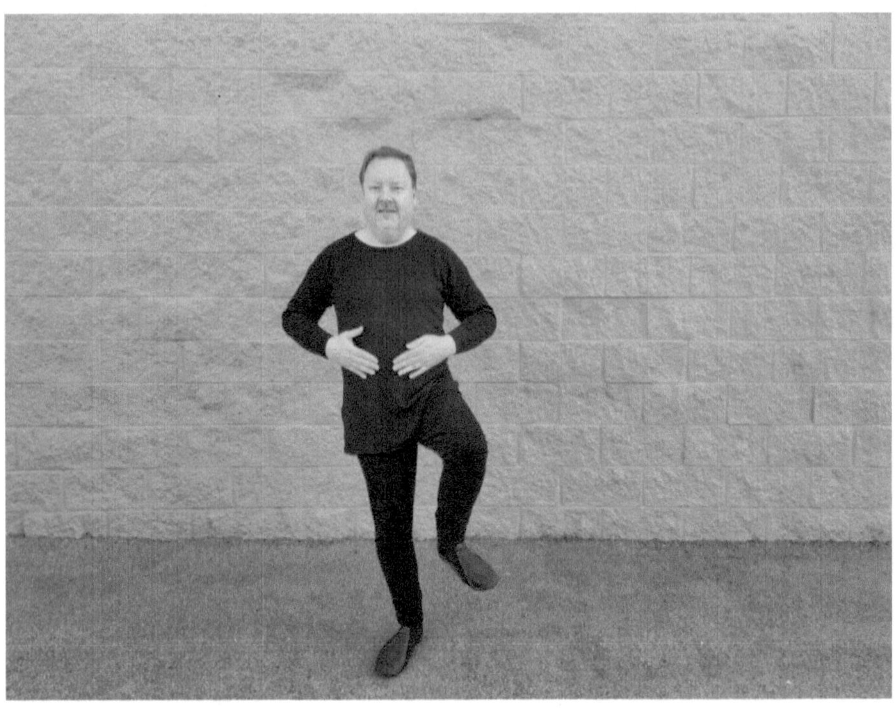

Figure 61 - Shift your full weight onto one leg, lift the other one as high as possible. Do this again with the other leg.

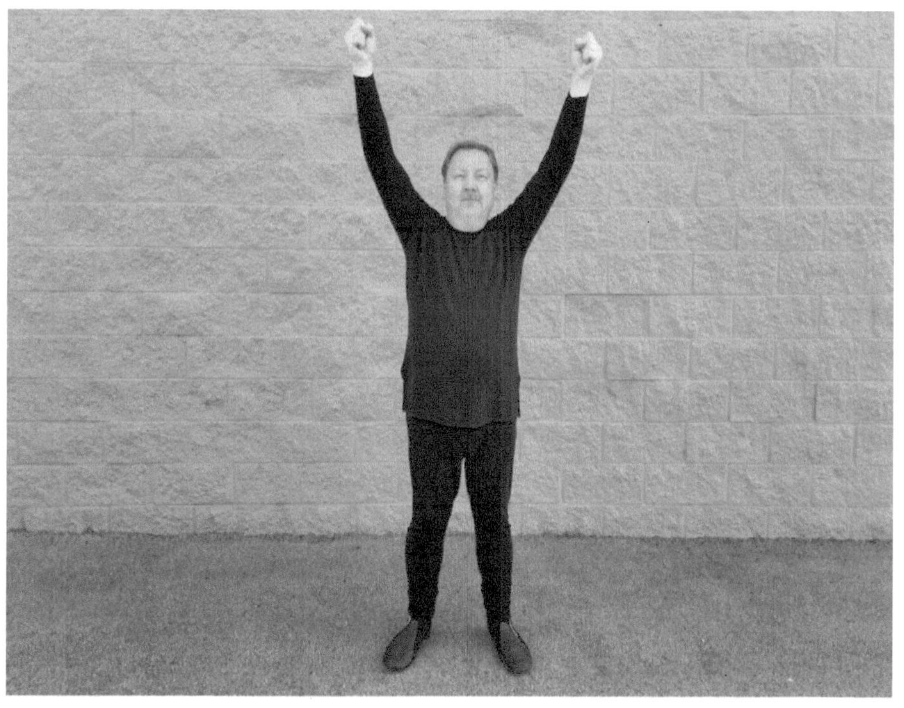

Figure 62 - Blessings from above. What will pour out in your life? What divine blessings are coming your way?

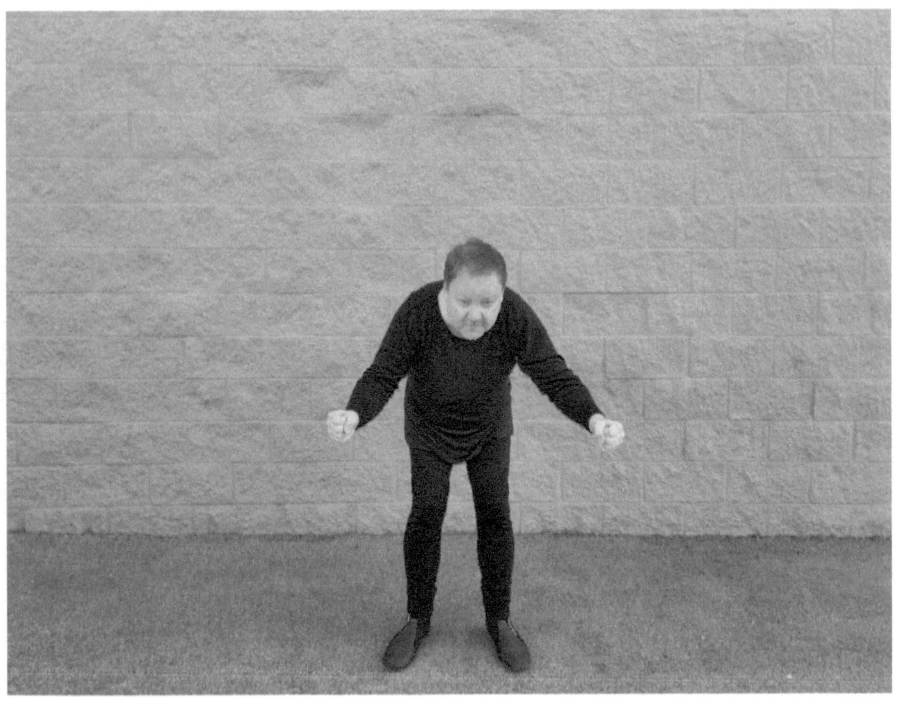

Figure 63 - Preparing to bend over with containers full of blessings from above.

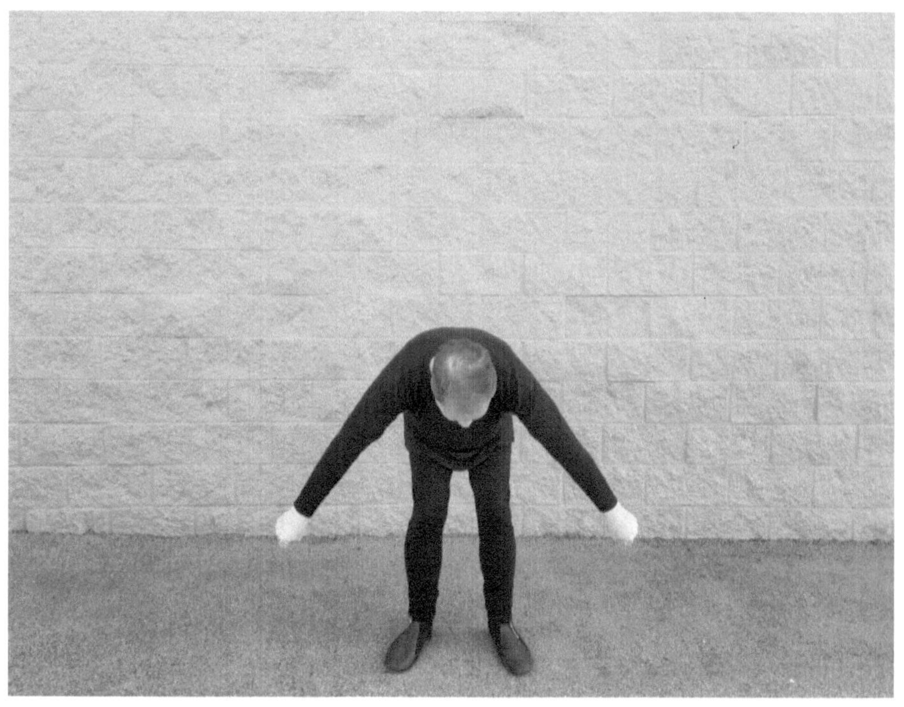

Figure 64 – Bending over to pour out all the blessings. As you pour, the containers get lighter and lighter, so your arms will lift back up to waist height.

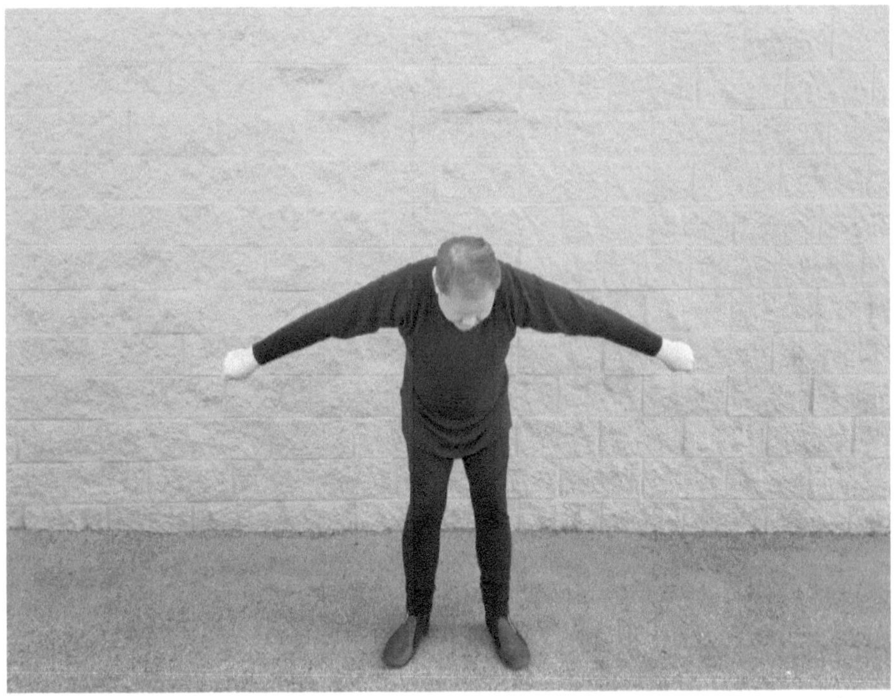

Figure 65 – As the containers poured out their contents, they became lighter and our arms lifted. We will be repeating this entire series of moves.

△△△

THE MOON

Chapter 19

Are you crazy as a loon, loony, or a lunatic?
Luna is the Latin word for moon.
You might just be moonstruck.

THE MOON is often a symbol of uncertainty, darkness, deception and instability. Often, it is a card of fear or terror. The card usually shows a dark scene or is set at night. Animals howl at two towers, and something rises from the deep waters below. The Man in the Moon, if shown, is often frowning down upon all. Altogether, it is an unsettling card.

But, just like so much of the symbology in Tarot, the meaning can also bring a beneficial, positive message. It can show you the need to stop, calm your animal nature, and create a bit of peace. Maybe it is a message, a warning that you are on a path that will lead to no good and you need to reevaluate.

We will physically interpret this card by raising our arms above our heads and form a circle, shaping the moon. Bring both arms straight down signifying the two towers. Then the hands cross in front of you at stomach level, signifying confusion.

Take a step back with your left foot first, followed by the right foot, and bend down while opening your arms. You reach down, and as you stand back up, cross your arms in front of you. This is another instance of the negative symbology of being "star-crossed" or having bad luck. As you continue to stand, you will uncross your arms and form the moon above your head again. Do the entire series of movements once more. You will not go to the home position, but transition directly into the next form.

<u>Movement/Energy Focus:</u>

Shoulders, Arms, Hands, Torso, Waist, Legs, Feet

<u>GO A LITTLE DEEPER:</u>

This is an opportunity for more deep stretching. As you reach up to form the moon, you can go up onto your toes. And as you lean down, you can extend your arms fully before bringing them together and crossing them. This will maximize the arm stretch. When you step back, you can make a shallow or deep step as you wish.

Remember the previous Tower card? Bad things just happen. But sometimes, we are our own worst enemy. We make the bad things happen. How many times have you looked back at something you said or did and thought, "if only…."

This card is a reminder to be mindful, be thoughtful. Think through your plans. Think through your dreams and goals. As you do this, be open to inspiration and forging new paths, making new plans. Because, as you stay open to new experiences and new ideas, they will show up. But if you are stubborn and refuse to budge from any path, then you may miss the better path that is in front of you.

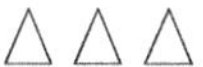

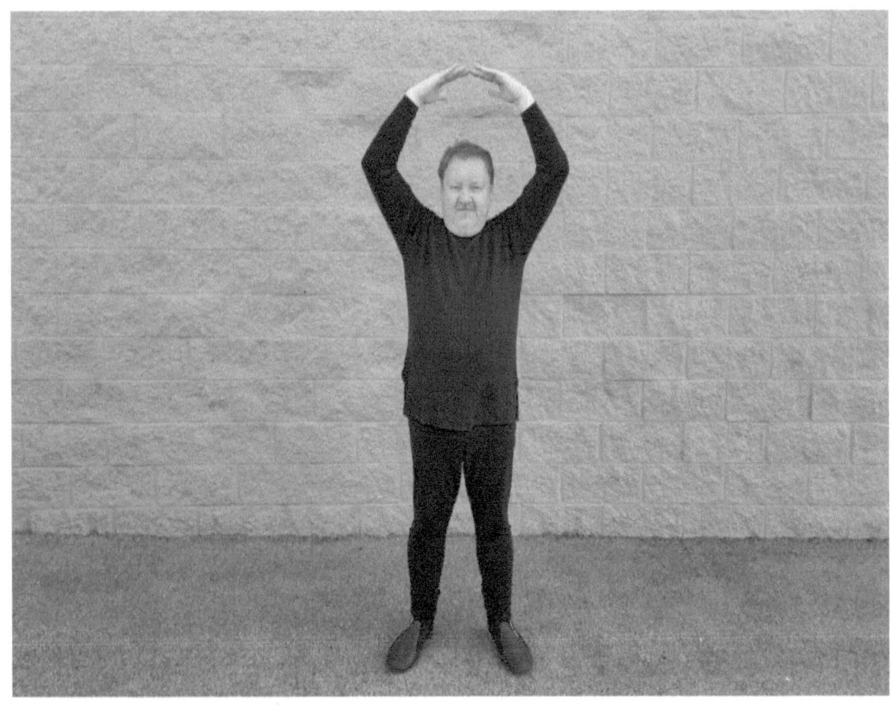

Figure 66 – Round out your arms and form the shape of the Moon.

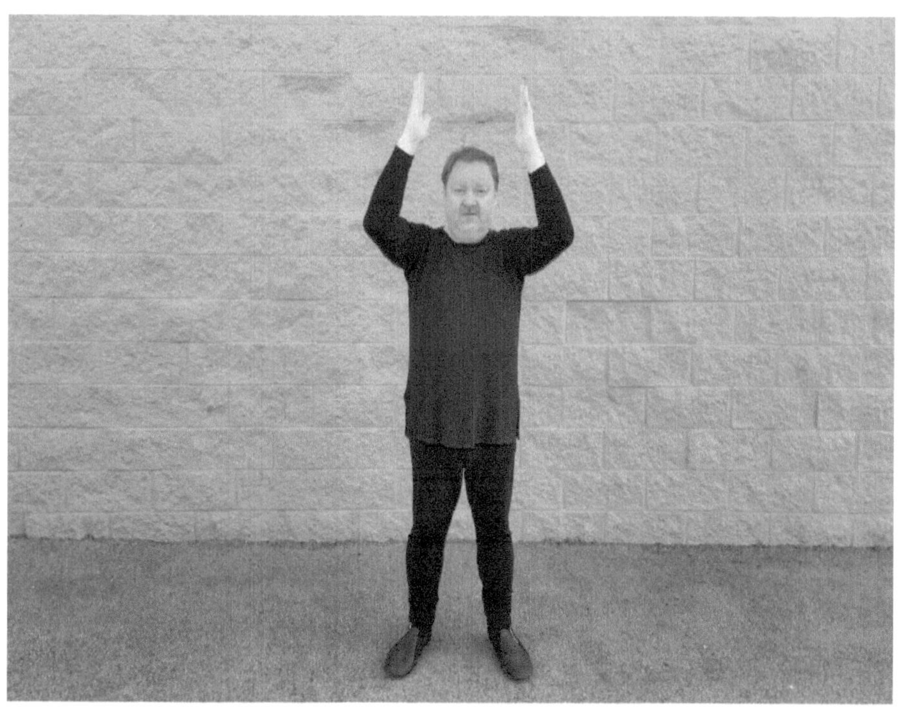

Figure 67 – Bringing the moon down, shaping two towers.

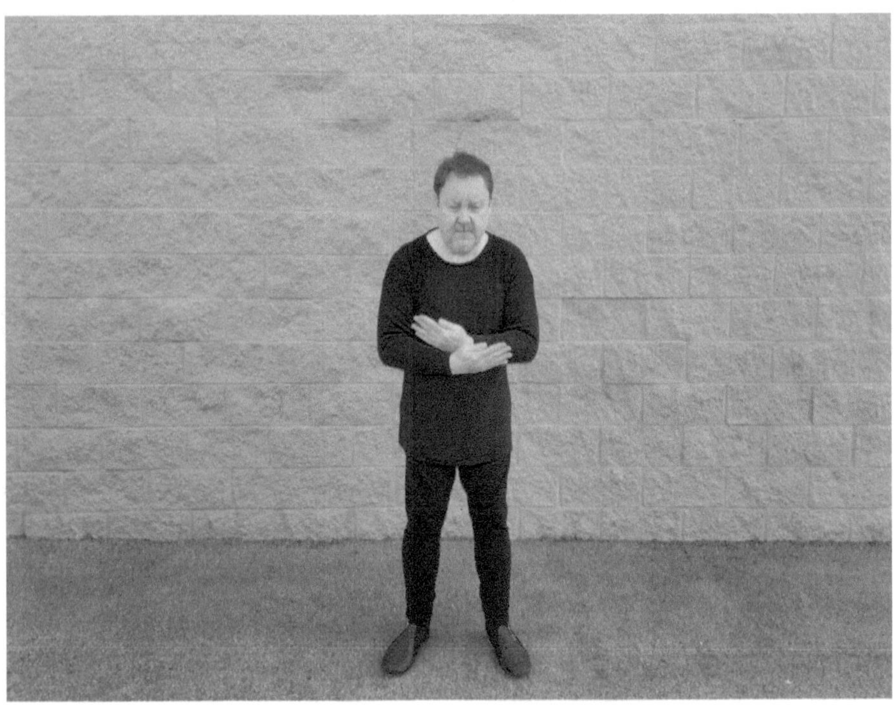

Figure 68 – As you continue to bring down the moon and the two towers, you will cross hands in front to symbolize confusion, the influence of negativity, or a dark matter.

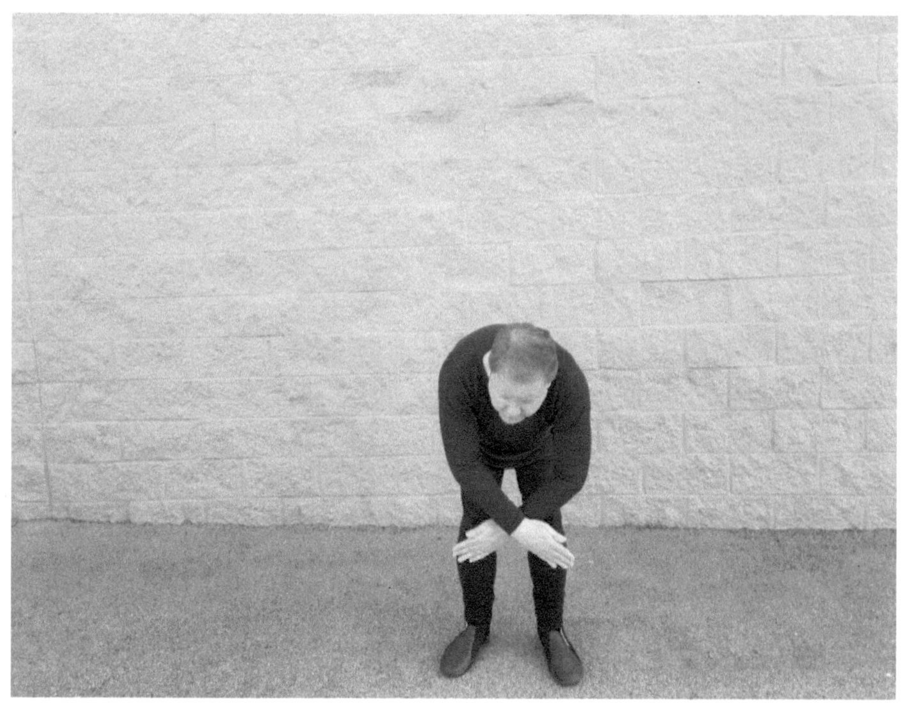

Figure 69 - Hands crossed low down on the body, as you reach down, crossing the arms, symbolizing something negative rising from the deep.

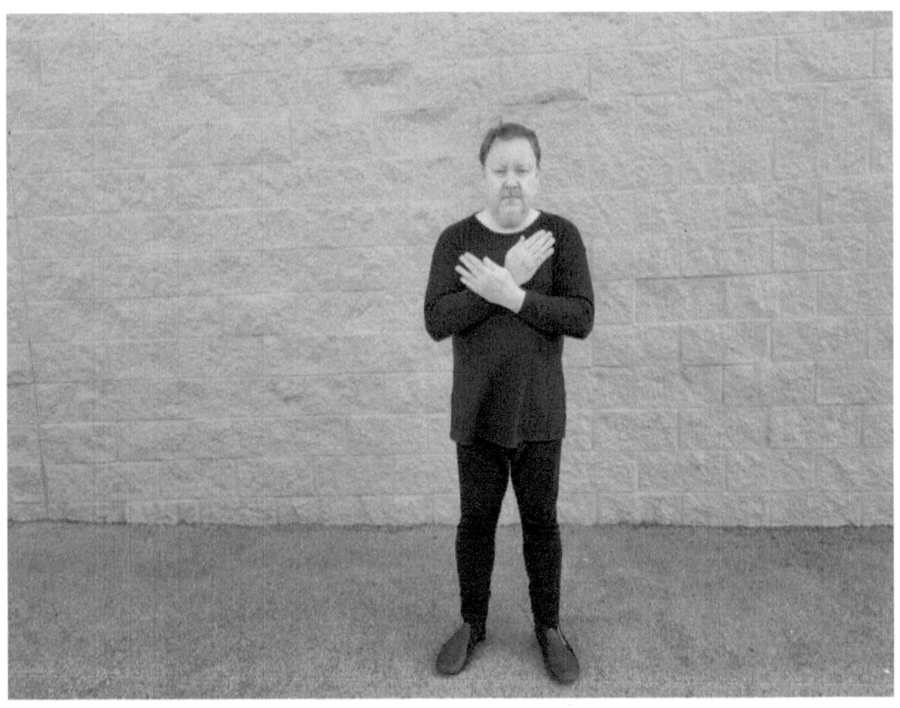

Figure 70 – Arms crossed as you rise, symbolizing a negative force that is crossing you. Your hands will continue up and over your head to shape the Moon again and repeat the series.

△△△

THE SUN

Chapter 20

Our Sun is a burning ball of gases.
Life on Earth exists because of our star.
Many billions of years from now,
life on Earth will die,
because a star cannot burn forever.

THE SUN is a supremely happy card with a happy scene. It is an image that usually shows innocence in the form of a child, often seen riding a white horse. There might be several naked children cavorting around naturally in the sun. It shines brightly above and sends blessings down onto the children below. Often, there are also sunflowers on the card, showing the way our sun literally brings forth life on our planet. Oh, how I love being out in the sun on a spring day; how about you? As I putter around with the flowers and plants on my back porch, it is like the whole world is right and exactly as it needs to be.

The sheer happiness of the Sun card contrasts with the unhappy nature of the previous Moon card. This card is the symbol of human mastery of the mind and the will over our baser, more negative urgings. The conscious mind (as indicated by the Sun) has become stronger than the unconscious (as indicated by the Moon.) We have mastered our thinking and mastered our interior fears.

Since you have just ended the Moon card, your arms will be in a circle above your head. Now, as the Sun, you will slowly swing your arms down and back up in a large arcing circle, three times. As you swing your arms down, you will also bend your knees in a squat and then rise back up as your arms go back up.

After the third circle, you will hold your arms up in the sunshine position and take one large step forward, with your right foot first, followed by your left foot, and into the bright sunshine.

Once you have taken that large step, you will hold the Sunshine position (the circle above your head) and begin wiggling your toes! Then begin wiggling your fingers. This is a symbolic representation of the shining, shimmering rays of the Sun. Begin a slow circle back down and to the home position, all while wiggling those fingers and toes. Remember to smile and breathe deeply as you go back to the home position.

<u>Movement/Energy Focus:</u>

Arms, Hands, Knees, Hips, Thighs, Fingers, Toes

GO A LITTLE DEEPER:

Make sure and wiggle all your toes and fingers at the end of this pose. One of the goals I had in Tarot-Chi ™ was for there to be an exercise system that literally exercised all the body, from head to toe. And here, we get to do just that. As you make the 3 large arcing circles, do it slowly and remember how good life truly is!

The balance of the Sun card is perfect after the darkness of some of the previous cards, like the Devil, the Tower and the Moon. But, without the darkness, you would never appreciate the light, right?

I grew up in the country. You never really know how dark it is unless you live in a rural area or you routinely get out and go camping. When you lean back and look at the night sky, the stars really stand out in the dark. This is the energy of the Sun card. Without the darkness of the night, we can't see the stars. Without the darkness of difficulties in life, we would not appreciate the good nearly as much.

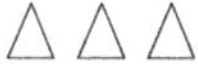

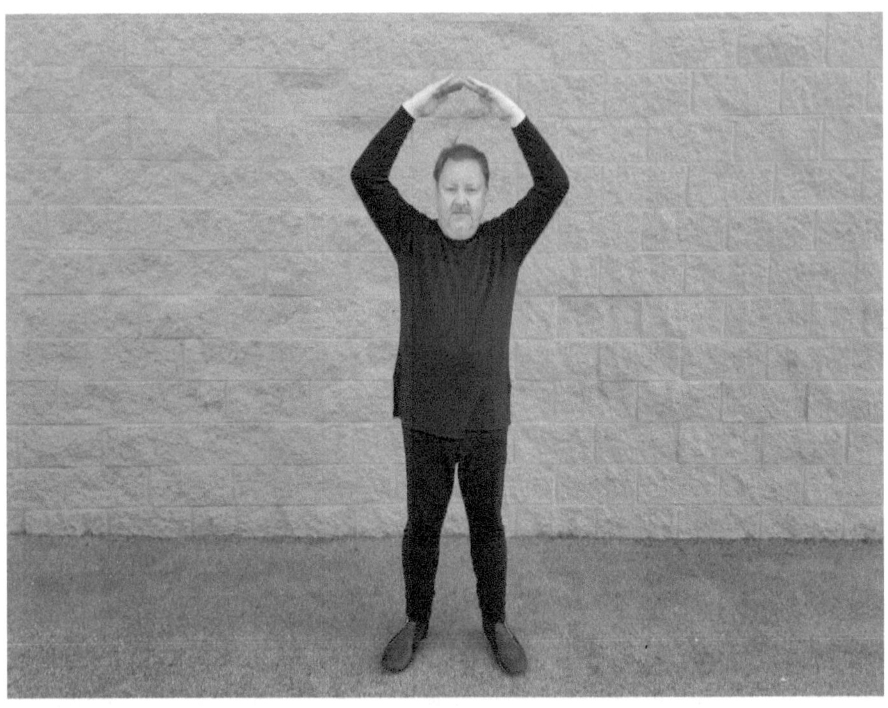

Figure 71 - Forming the shape of the Sun. Yes, it looks just like the Moon, but the energy and intent are very different.

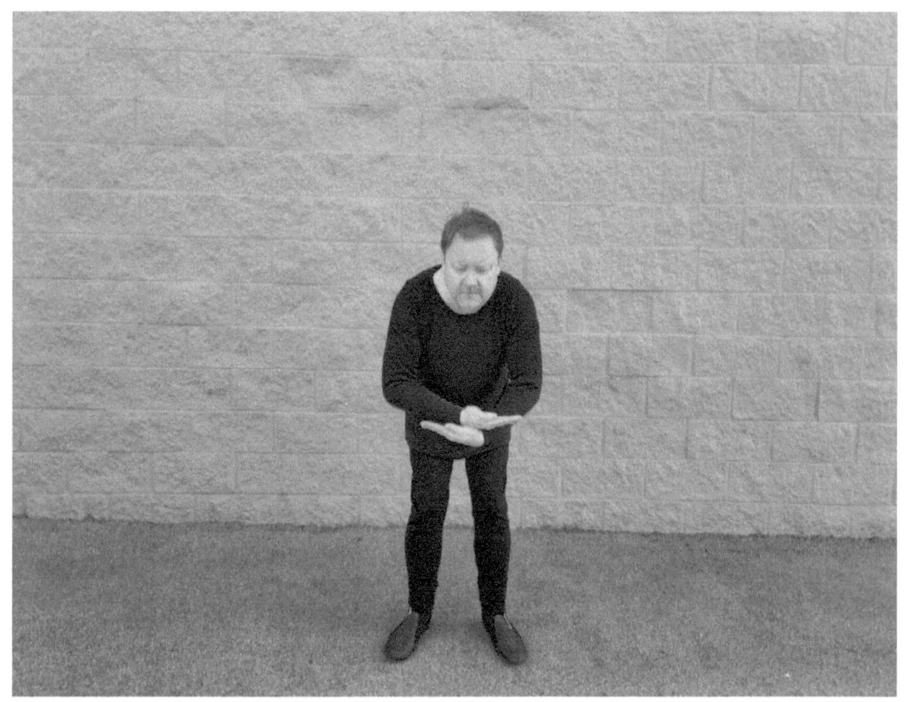

Figure 72– Bend down and then back up 3 times, swinging your arms in a big arc. The hands do not cross like in the Moon series, but meet at the bottom before swinging back up again.

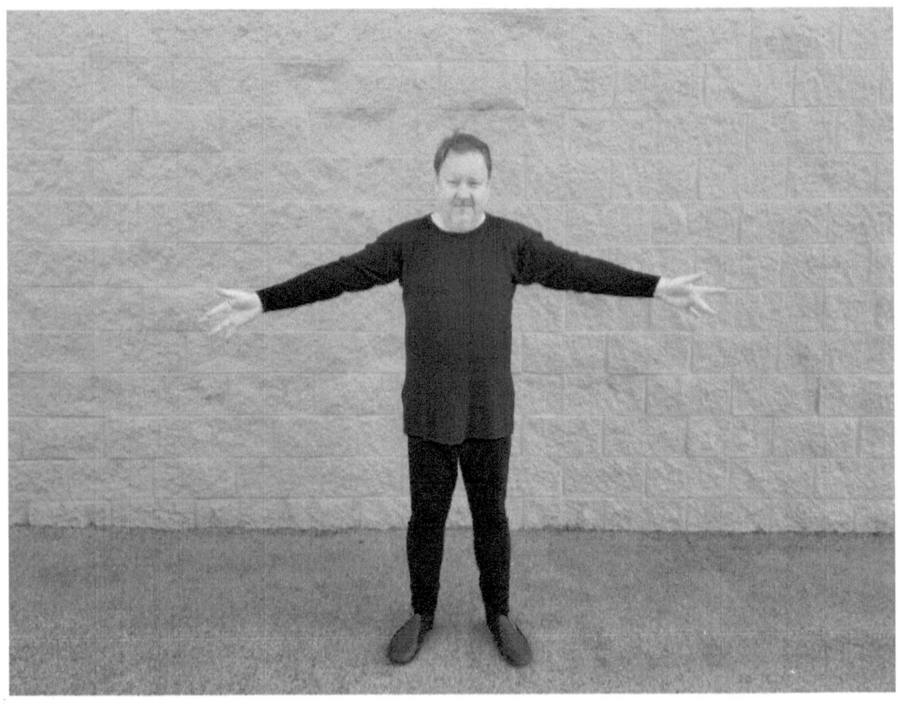

Figure 73 - After forming the Sun 3 times, you will take a huge step into the light, and then begin wiggling your toes. Arc your arms down once more, wiggling your fingers to symbolize the Sun's rays.

△△△

JUDGEMENT

Chapter 21

No one else is living your life.
No one else has suffered your pains.
No one else knows your dreams.
No one else can judge your actions.

JUDGEMENT day is here! This card usually shows an angel blowing a great trumpet, at which dead people happily rise from coffins. It shows that last reckoning when you must answer to a higher power for your wrongdoing and sins, or get rewarded for your kindness and generosity. All sorts of human cultures, from ancient Egypt to the Maya, have had this idea of judgement of the soul. Although, the happiest resurrected people are probably those who believe they will not be judged too harshly.

We will begin by stepping to the right, holding the right hand up to the right ear as if you might have heard a trumpet sound. Go back to center and do the motion on the left side. Back to center.

Once again, you will step to the right and then the left, only this time, as you step out, you will lean and stretch out as far as possible with your right hand. Repeat with the left side and the left hand. During the second set of these poses, you will lean forward onto the front leg as you lift the heel of the back foot. Your palm can be up or it can be down, either way is fine.

Once you come back to the center position, lean down from the waist as far as you can. You can bend the knees if needed, or keep your knees straight if you can. Extend your arms behind you. You will make a sweeping motion, with palms up lifting your hands and body up from the ground and all the way to the heavens, twisting your hands outward as you go up. As your hands rise to the skies, look upward. This is a good stretch for your neck, too. You will not go back to the home position, but will transition directly to the next form.

Movement/Energy Focus:

Legs, Knees, Feet, Arms, Waist, Torso, Hands

GO A LITTLE DEEPER:

Lots of opportunities in this series of poses for you to get in some extra stretching, flexing and movement. When you step to the left and right, you can make that as shallow or deep as you choose. During that section of the poses, your arm will be outstretched. You can go palm up or palm down. With palm up, you are aligned more with asking and receiving mercy. With palms down, you are more aligned with projecting a sense of mastery and self-empowerment. Some days, I feel like I truly need the palm up handout; but other days I'm like, "Nope, I got this!" Whichever feels best to you is what you should do.

Let's talk a moment about judgement; not divine, but human. I was taught that you do not judge others. I still live by that rule. You never know what someone else is going through, so my basic rule is to give everyone a pass with grace. If someone is rude to me, well, I chalk it up to them having a bad day, year or life. I do not let it get to me. I do not judge others' actions and reactions. They must judge themselves.

But the idea of grace and non-judgement only goes so far. I DO make a judgement for myself as to whether I will allow someone else's actions and reactions to impact my life further. If someone is awful to me, I do not judge them. But I also do not allow them the opportunity to screw with me again. I learned this the hard way. I have fewer closer friends now, but my life is a lot more peaceful.

Don't take shit from anyone. Be you. Be fiercely you! That is a judgement call that you can 100% make.

△△△

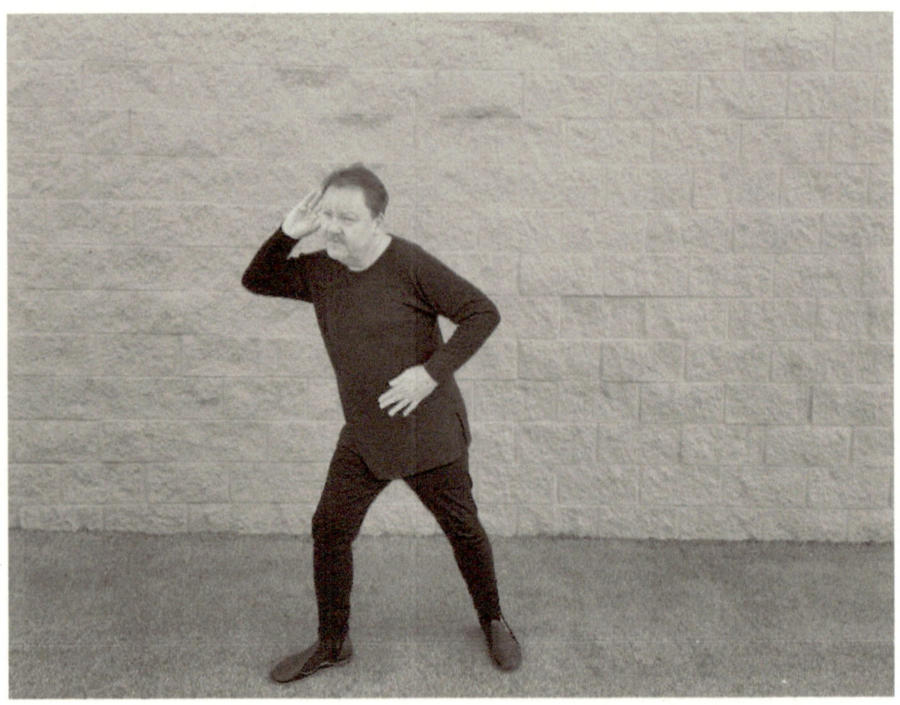

Figure 74 - What do you hear? It is the trumpet blast of judgement. Step to the left and listen. Then step to the right and listen.

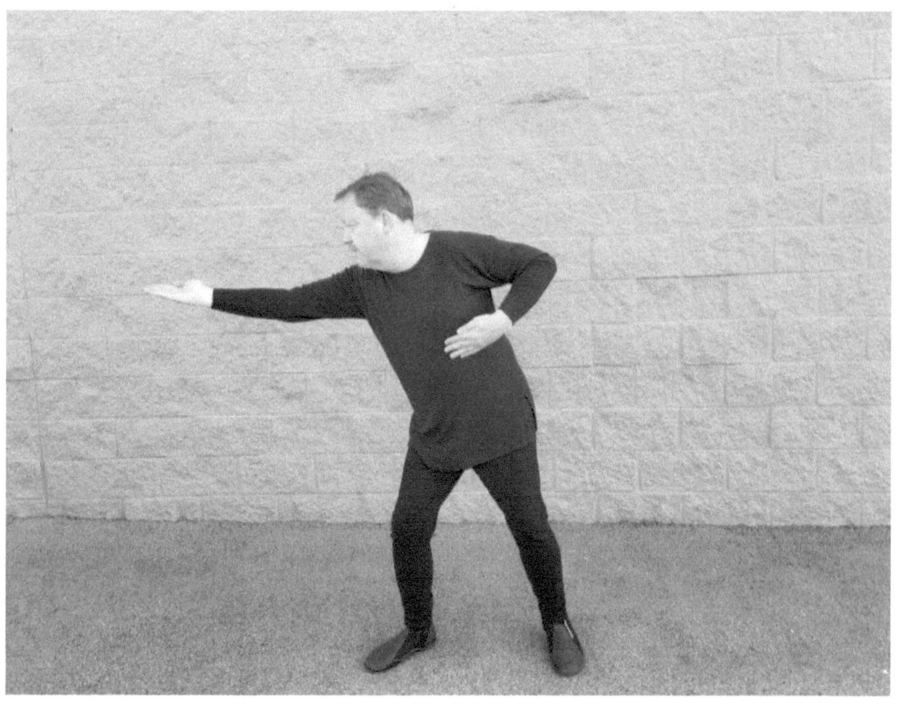

Figure 75 - A nice stretch as we look to find the source of the sound. Palms can be up or down.

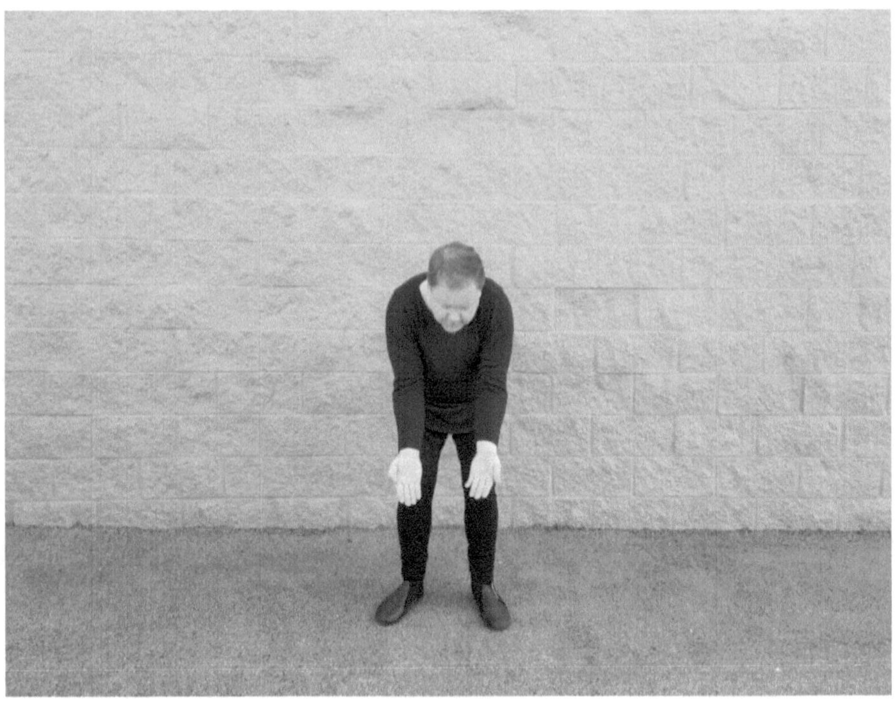

Figure 76 - All rise for judgement! You swing your arms back behind you and then forward in a sweeping motion all the way up above your head.

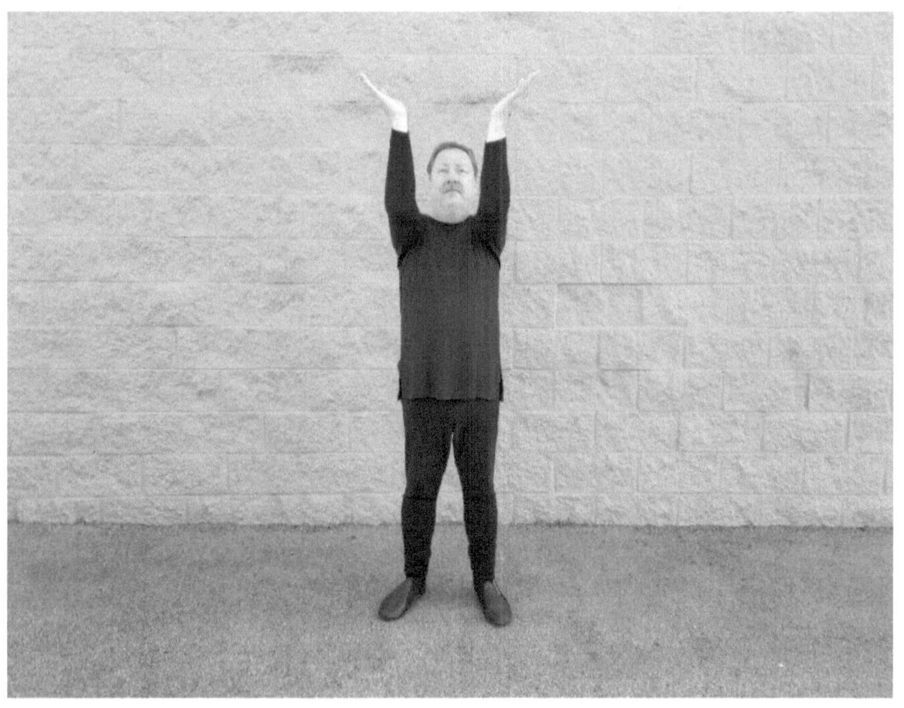

Figure 77 – As you complete the sweeping motion, you will raise your hands to the heavens.

△△△

THE WORLD

Chapter 22

Do not underestimate your power to change the world - not the huge world filled with everyone, but the little world of your family and friends.

THE WORLD is the summation of all things, the symbology of the final end of it all. In some decks, this card has overt Christian symbolism, with images straight out of the Book of Revelations. There are often people and beasts on the card, or astrological symbols. Later decks are more likely to avoid religious symbolism and focus instead on the natural world or even the world beyond our Earth, the Universe.

Whatever the symbolism, this is the end of the whole Tarot cycle that began with The Fool. And it is the indication that life is circular, that it keeps repeating, that each end is just another beginning. We see this in nature, as decay leads to new growth. It is the same with people. You have seen this same idea presented throughout Tarot-Chi™ as endings become beginnings.

This final series of movements will remind you of the halfway mark in Tarot-Chi with The Wheel of Fortune card. Clasp both hands together above your head, and imagine you are holding a huge marker or pen. Step back with your right foot and pivot on your left heel. You are now facing a different direction. Beginning at the top, you will scribe a full circle, swinging your arms to the right. As you go down, bend your knees. Then as you swing your arms to the left, stand back up and bring your left foot back beside your right foot and close the circle.

You are now ready to start a new circle by putting your right foot behind you and pivoting on your left heel. You will make this full circle four times, each time facing another of the four directions. At each direction, you can focus on that classic element – Earth in the North, Air in the East, Fire in the South, and Water in the West. When you make the last pivot and the last circle, and have brought your feet together, then allow your arms to slowly circle back down and place them on your stomach in the home position.

Close your eyes, and we will end the same way we began. Breathe in through your nose, hold it, and then breathe out through your mouth. Do this three times. And then open your eyes.

<u>Movement/Energy Focus:</u>

Arms, Shoulders, Hands, Torso, Waist, Legs, Feet

GO A LITTLE DEEPER:

At this point, we are done with the entire Tarot-Chi ™ cycle. At this moment, you are back in the home position where everything began. Your hands are on your stomach. You are breathing deeply. You have spent the last 11-12 minutes stretching every bit of your body, literally from your head to your toes. You have received energy from the Earth and from Heaven above. Well done!

As I make the circles and greet the four directions, I mentally tally up the blessings from each. I will speak out loud and say, "Thank you fire, for warming my home." And I will be thankful to each of the elements of the four directions for what they are bringing to me. Yes, honoring the four directions is a very old-fashioned idea; but you will find it is still done in First Nations and Native American cultures throughout North America, from Canada to Mexico.

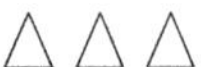

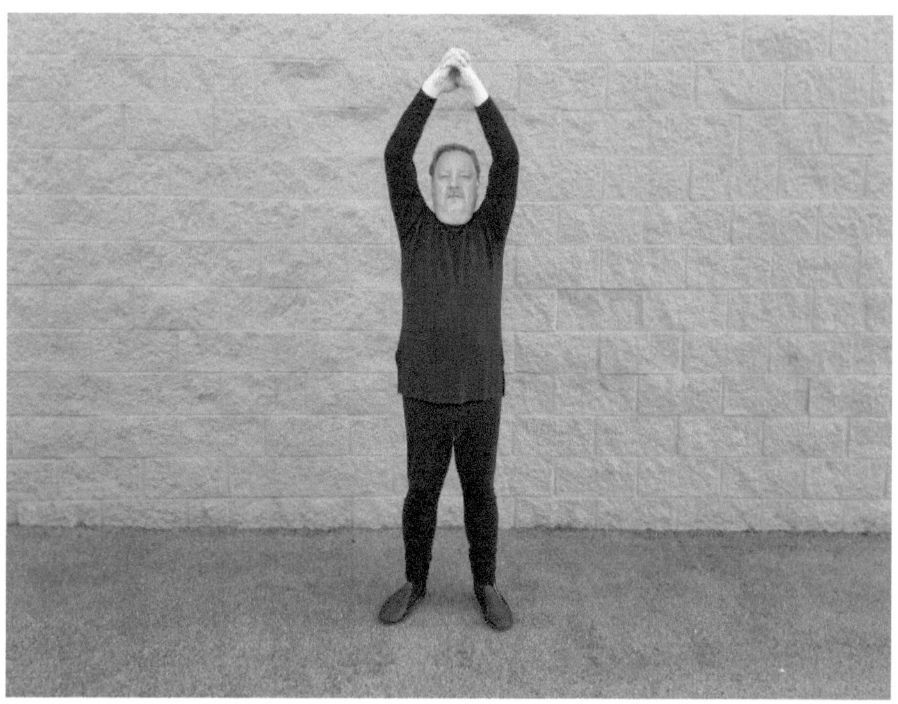

Figure 78 – For the last card and series of poses, this beginning position is similar to the Wheel of Fortune at the halfway mark in Tarot-Chi ™

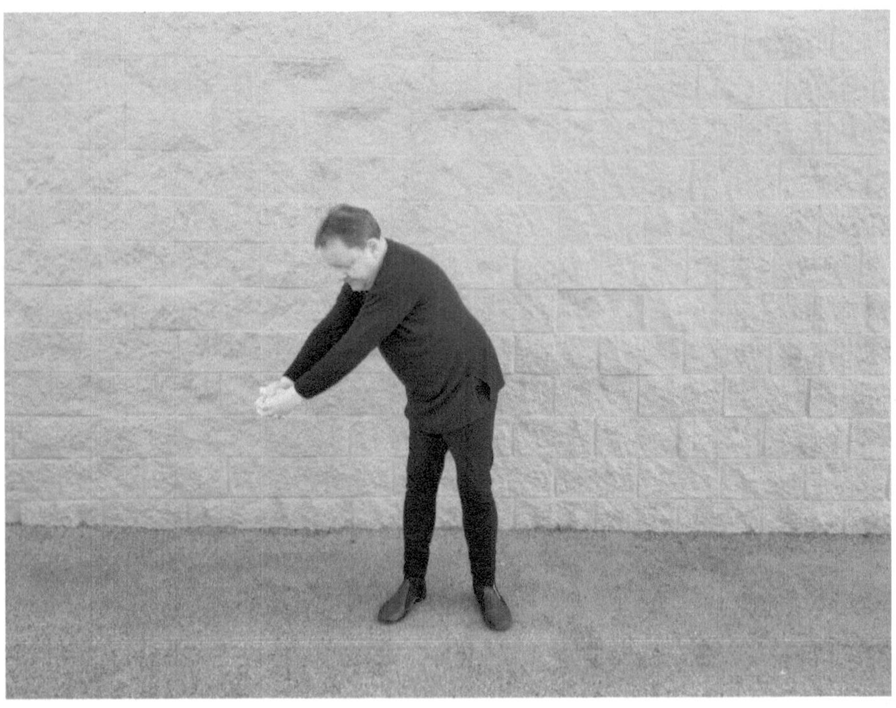

Figure 79 – Keeping your arms extended and hands clasped, rotate to the right as you create a circle with your hands and arms.

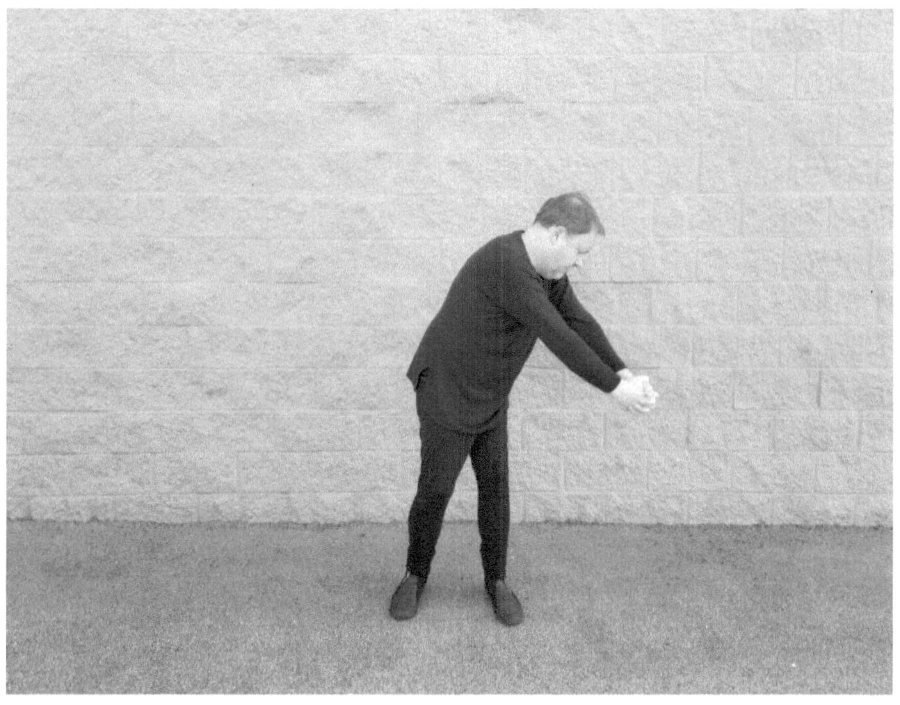

Figure 80 - Rotation to the left as you close the circle. Remember to repeat this four times, each time facing one of the four directions.

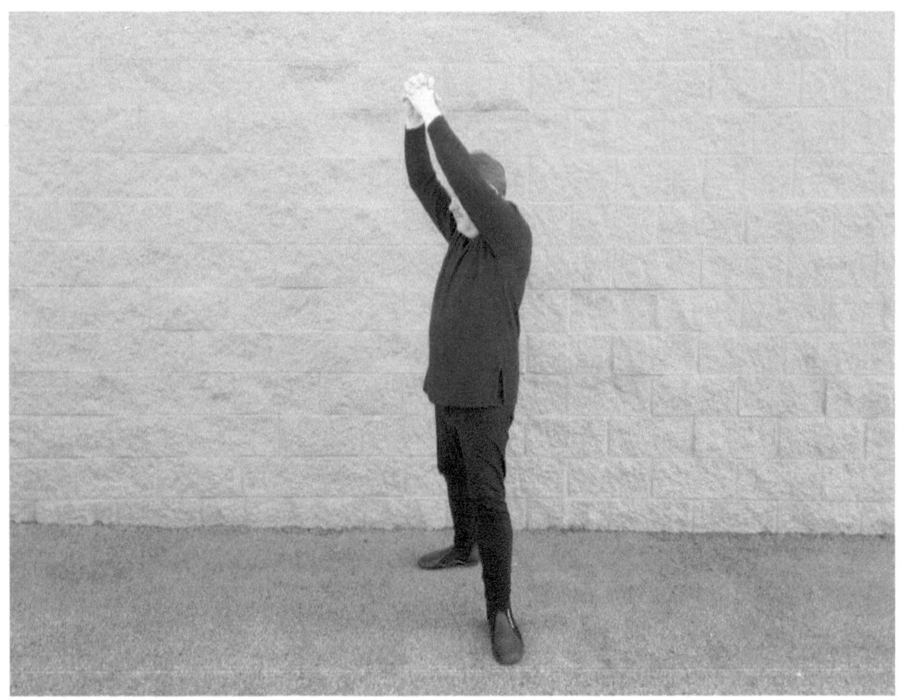

Figure 81 – Pivot and face each direction as you make a circle with your hands. You will bring your feet together as you finish scribing the circle in that direction before pivoting to the next direction.

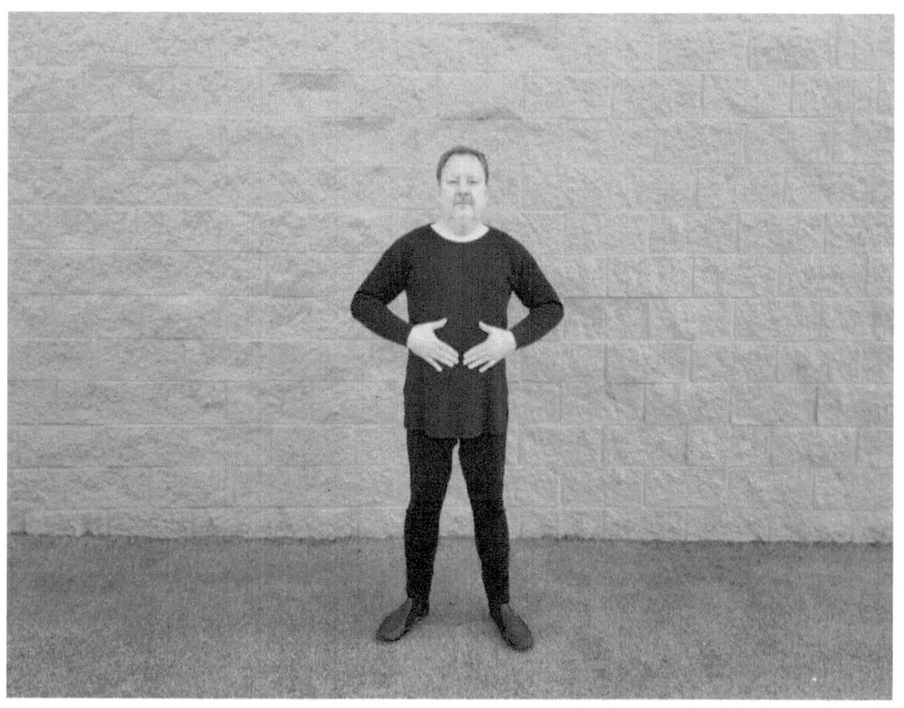

Figure 82 - And the final Home position! Close your eyes, take three deep breaths, and then you are done.

△ △ △

FINAL THOUGHTS

Chapter 23

"If we shadows have offended, think but this and all is mended, that you have but slumber'd here. And this weak and idle theme, no more yielding but a dream." – Shakespeare's Puck from A Midsummer Night's Dream

TAROT-CHI ™ is fun! As you finish up each session, make sure and rehydrate. Go get a drink of water and wash your hands. This is for more than just hydration - it also signifies a return to the here and now, an end of the flow of energy and the end of your session.

It's a funny thing about exercise; I always hate to get started, but I'm upset when it is over! So much in life is like that, right? We have a goal or a task and we put it off, dreading it. Then, once we finally start, we find that it isn't all that bad, and that hey, it's actually kind of fun!

The creation of Tarot-Chi ™ was that way for me. It seemed like a daunting task at first. But the process really did seem to fall into place. It is now a part of my daily routine, and I have received so many blessings because of it. Anytime that you can add an easy exercise routine to your daily life, then you are going to reap some serious benefits. But the beauty of this is that it is not just physical. The mental and psychological benefits stack up, too. I truly hope Tarot-Chi ™ brings blessings and benefits to you throughout your life, too.

I hope you have enjoyed learning this system. And I hope that once you learn it you will continue. This is one of those exercise systems that will bring more benefit the more you practice it. It only takes 11 or so minutes to complete, and yet I believe it can be a powerful system to help your body heal naturally, along with helping your mind and spirit heal.

The motivation to create this system might surprise you. Let me tell you a quick story about my last husband, David. He was a Wushu master. He passed away several years ago at the age of 46. We had been married for only 11 months. But during that short time, he shared some wonderful stories of the martial art that he loved and how it had changed his life. (We had known each other for 17 years.) He specifically taught me a breathing technique that I used during the terrible waves of grief that followed his death. It is a bittersweet irony that he had such a positive impact on me even after he was gone.

After we married, he encouraged me to try a martial art of my own. I had been in a serious car wreck before we married and I was not in the best of health. He encouraged me to try Tai Chi, thinking it would be gentle and kind for my wounded body. It was, but I still was not able to commit to the system. It just did not speak to me. It just did not make a connection with my spirit.

When David asked me why, I told him about the way I would always see the Tarot cards in my mind when I was practicing Tai Chi. I am a daughter of the Western world; the ideas and mysticism of the West make more sense to me. He casually mentioned that it was too bad there wasn't an exercise system based on the Tarot instead. It was just a simple comment, and yet, after he died, I remembered it. Through the years, I began looking for and seeing more of the connections and associations that became the basis of Tarot-Chi ™.

What I was NOT looking for during that time was love, and yet my new husband, Mark, casually walked into my life. He was not a martial arts master, but he had always loved the imagery of the Tarot. When I told him about my idea for Tarot-Chi ™, he absolutely loved it! His influence was tremendous in the months where I was creating this system. And he is usually right beside me each day when I exercise.

I am now stronger physically and mentally than I have ever been. Tarot-Chi ™ has helped me in so many ways. My core is stronger which has helped with my chronic back pain. My stamina has increased, along with improved flexibility and balance. Along the way, my spiritual and emotional life has improved. I believe this can happen for you, too. The psychological journey you can take with Tarot-Chi ™ can be just as powerful as the physical one.

Once you learn the physical system, then those movements become automatic in what martial arts practitioners call "muscle memory." As you do the movements and poses that are now in your body's muscle memory, your mind is able to focus on healing old thoughts and emotions that are no longer beneficial for you.

Once you learn Tarot-Chi ™ you can then create the perfect associations with each movement for your emotional and psychological needs. I recommend you focus on positive imagery you want to associate with each card and the poses. Remember the recommendation I had for going deeper with The Lovers card? I always imagine that positive blessing are coming to me and my spouse. I have attuned my physical body and emotional/spiritual mind to focus on that.

When I follow through with the movements associated with The Devil card, I focus on what areas in my life need to be released. I have never been addicted to drugs, but I have struggled with food addiction. I focus on releasing and healing that part of my life when I release the chained captives of The Devil card.

Create the imagery with each card to bring in what you need and banish what you don't. Take my suggestions and then go create the images and associations that work for you. Hope and healing can be yours, just sometimes you have to create it for yourself. I have been incredibly blessed by this system, in body, mind and spirit. I am excited to share this journey with you and hope you will be blessed for the rest of your life, too!

ABOUT THE AUTHOR

Shanna and her husband, Mark, live in Oklahoma. She has written several books, and has many more in the works. As a trauma survivor, her focus is on helping others. And as a paranormal experiencer, she tells fantastic true stories about her mysterious life.

Visit https://www.ShannaWarner.com for links to her books. Sign up for the blog and newsletter while you are there. She is the author of *Easy Stress Solutions: How to Meditate Like a Master, Banish Anxiety and Kick Depression to the Curb* and also *Ghost Encounters: 13 True Tales of the Supernatural.*

Shanna is available for in-person and video conferences, speaking engagements and expos. Please request a media kit and information regarding speaker's fees at: chatwithshanna@gmail.com. Please have an idea regarding venue size and attendance.

WORK WITH US

Tarot-Chi ™ is a registered trademark with the US Patent and Trade Office. You cannot use the name, trademark or any of the related intellectual property without permission. You cannot start classes or teach the system without training and authorization. (And if you do, that is some really bad karma. And I know you don't want that!) We want this program to be successful for as many people as possible and we want it to be beneficial and authentic. If you are interested in becoming a Certified Tarot-Chi ™ Instructor, please go to **https://www.Tarot-Chi.com** and fill out the contact form. As a certified instructor, you can charge a small access fee for classes and create a second stream of income for yourself, similar to the way martial arts or yoga classes work. We will certify only 1 instructor per city or zip code, and will support you with training and marketing materials as you begin sharing and teaching this system. We look forward to partnering with you!

- Shanna and Mark Warner

THE END

Like all endings, this is really just another BEGINNING.
Whatever happens for you now, I hope it is something great!

www.ingramcontent.com/pod-product-compliance
Lightning Source LLC
LaVergne TN
LVHW090951080826
845145LV00003B/973

* 9 7 8 1 9 5 3 0 9 8 0 7 8 *